I Can't Remember Me

I Can't Remember Me:

Recovery after traumatic brain injury

Judy Martin-Urban
with
Courtney Martin Larson

I CAN'T REMEMBER ME:

RECOVERY AFTER TRAUMATIC BRAIN INJURY

Judy Martin-Urban
with
Courtney Martin Larson

Cover: Michael Qualben
Copyright © 2006 by Judy Martin-Urban and
Courtney Martin Larson
Bear Sculpture: Charles Schiefer Permission
First Printing 2006
Printed in the United States of America

Published by
LangMarc Publishing
P.O. Box 90488
Austin Texas 78709-0488

Library in Congress Control Number: 2006922015

ISBN: 1-880292-793

DEDICATED TO THE MEMORY OF

ZACHARY PARIS

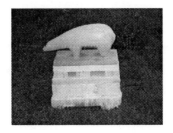

AND

TO ALL PEOPLE WITH DISABILITIES

The marvelous richness of human experience
would lose something of rewarding joy if
there were not limitations to overcome.
The hilltop hour would not be half so wonderful
if there were no dark valleys to traverse.

—Helen Keller

CONTENTS

ACKNOWLEDGMENTS

I thank my family who stood behind me throughout everything. Special thanks go to my husband, Conrad, for just being there. Our blended children and grandchildren deserve more credit than I can say, for without their support, things would have been much harder. Gratitude also goes to our extended family, including my siblings and their families, Conrad's parents (now deceased), his sister and family and numerous friends and acquaintances.

Thanks to the people at my workplace, Aegis Women's Healthcare, and our church, Saint Thomas Lutheran, both in Bloomington, Indiana, who gave love of hearts abundant. Deep thanks go to my prayer partner at that time, Shari Rogge-Fiddler. God knew I would need her when He sent her my way.

I thank the members of my Muncie Writing Group for their faith and encouragement.

Sincere thanks also go to our publisher, LangMarc Publishing.

Judy Martin-Urban

I want to thank my husband Jerry, who is my most loyal friend and was my supporter throughout this experience. He has helped me to make the progress that I have.

Christina remains the light of my life, and I thank her for being who she is, a wonderfully strong daughter and person. She gives me reason to live.

I thank God for giving me back my life and for His miraculous healing of my body.

To my Mother and to the rest of my family I say thank you for your faith and your love.

Courtney Martin Larson

INTRODUCTION

My daughter and I offer a personal view into windows of our lives in hopes that those of you suffering grief and loss will find common threads of understanding and be helped in recovery from your grief. These words had to be written as part of our healing from our deep grief. We have recovered and now own the journey as part of our selves.

Our words are simple and speak from our hearts. Our story begins with the car accident, because the accident is where my grandson died and where tragedy created a new woman from the daughter I had borne, raised, and relinquished.

Tragedy happens in every life and vulnerability follows. The ensuing grief is a universal phenomenon without respecter of person. Our culture teaches us very little in how to get through our grief. If you're like we are, books personalizing how individuals have triumphed over their challenges remain most memorable.

Go to your fear. This is where you will find your courage.

Judy Martin-Urban, Mother

CHAPTER ONE

CALL IN THE NIGHT

Our telephone clamored like an alarm clock that night, October 7, 1997, just as I was falling into bed after a strenuous workday. Our son-in-law Jerry, choking and sobbing, cried that Courtney and Zachary had been involved in a car accident and were being life-lined to a hospital in Cincinnati, Ohio. He knew only that it was a one-car crash and that Christina, Courtney's daughter, had not been with them. Courtney is my daughter; Zachary is my six-year-old grandson.

My husband, Conrad, and I lived three hours from Cincinnati; we left immediately. In the dark of the night, we drove through one small town after another. It was during one of these subconscious blurs that I, with tears flowing, said to Conrad, "Zachary is gone." My heart knew he had died. Conrad silently touched my knee as pain engulfed me.

Courtney is my oldest daughter and, like many firstborns, had challenged her father, now deceased, and me. She had done everything early, including it seemed, growing up. At age nineteen, after only one year of college, she became a single mother of lovely little Christina. She worked hard to be independent and to provide for her daughter.

Eventually, she fell in love and married Art Paris, then a college student. Art adopted Christina, and later Zachary was born. The marriage lasted four years.

Jerry Larson and Courtney had been married a year when the accident occurred. Courtney had managed to finish the college degree begun at age eighteen. She and Jerry had worked to create a new and blended family. Jerry has four older children.

As we drove the miles that night, vivid memories raced through my mind. Courtney had made several fateful decisions in her young life.

At the hospital, we were met by a distraught Jerry, struggling vainly for control, and by a frightened 12-year-old Christina, who was silent as stone and, I was sure, in shock. Christina had decided at the last minute not to go to the store with Courtney and Zachary.

I held onto Christina. Words could not come. I gasped at the sight of Courtney and called her name, but I was answered by the hiss of machinery. We were told she was in a deep coma and was on life support from a traumatic brain injury. She was engulfed with tubes, machines, lights, and alarms. She looked so frightening and so sick that I almost panicked. They told us that her comatose state was further deepened with powerful medications given in an effort to decrease swelling in her brain and to prevent her from having a seizure. She had a tracheotomy, was on a ventilator, and had a catheter into her skull to monitor pressure on her brain. She wore a neck collar. She had multiple breaks in her pelvis, torn left knee ligaments, as well as compound breaks in the tibia and fibula of her left leg. Multiple contusions and abrasions covered her body, but, incredibly, her face had been spared.

It was hard to believe what I was seeing. Was this really my daughter Courtney?

My mind raced in a thousand directions with questions, but soon slammed into a brick wall. There would be no answers for a long time, if ever. I looked from Jerry to Christina. They were both pale and quiet.

She's going to die. My daughter's going to die. I could not quiet the thoughts.

It seemed impossible. I grabbed Christina and Jerry and held them tight. We said little, too numbed to cry. We stood close, trying to gain strength from one another. Conrad's strong arms encircled me.

Courtney's life was in question. If it had not been for the aggressive and competent medical and nursing teams at the University Hospital Surgical Trauma Intensive Care Unit, I believe she would have died. Her injuries were so severe that, by medical standards, she should have died.

On Courtney's admission to the hospital, her Glasco Coma Scale had been a four; 15 is optimum. Doctors use this scale to rank the extent of injury and chances of recovery. This scale of 3-15 involves testing three areas: eye opening, best verbal response, and best motor response. The higher the score the better the prognosis, and the lower the score the less chance there is for recovery. She was paralyzed and unresponsive. At one point, her Glasco score dropped to a three. Things did not look good.

Many of her injuries and diagnoses were intimidating, and I am glad we weren't fully aware of everything at the time. As a health care provider, I had been around hospitals and many sick people, but all I could see was my daughter hooked up to every imaginable kind of tube and machine. I began to ache with knowing what was to come.

We were told she had a closed head injury with a fracture at the base of her skull. There was a question whether she had a brain stem injury, which, if true, would definitely have made the rest of her life a vegetative state. They mentioned her multiple pelvic fractures, including a broken back. They were unsure if her neck was broken, but they were taking precautions by using the collar. Later we were told she did not have a brain stem injury or a broken neck. Our relief was immense, but waiting for that information had been agonizing.

After seeing Courtney, I thought I would be more prepared to see Zachary, but I wasn't. The shock was just as great and the pain just as real. He was also surrounded by life support machines but without as many other attachments. He had suffered an axonal head trauma or basically also a traumatic brain injury. Other than a few new scratches, his little body looked perfectly whole, just as if he were sleeping. But I knew he was gone. He was just being sustained until all could gather. He was just a small child, and small children aren't supposed to die. A part of me also died in that room with Zachary that night. I look forward to someday reclaiming that part of me that died that night.

Children's Hospital is connected to University Hospital by an underground tunnel. We made our way through the tunnel and went from bedside to bedside throughout the night. This was the longest and darkest night. All that mattered to any of us was that they were going to live. I kept my thoughts about Zachary to myself.

Courtney and Zachary each had been wearing seatbelts, but the tragedy was compounded by the fact that Courtney had alcohol and marijuana in her bloodstream. Learning this information was unbearable.

The car she had been driving was new to her and much larger than the car she usually drove. The road was curvy and the weather had been damp. According to witnesses, she had been driving fast when she lost control, went off the road and hit head on a large tree in a farmer's yard. It had taken 45 minutes to extricate her from the car.

Five years later, Courtney said she vaguely remembers swerving to avoid the oncoming car. It took that long for any memory of the accident to return. We'll never know whether she was distracted by Zachary, or what actually did happen, but the accident changed lives forever.

I called Zachary's dad and stepmother, Art and Dawn Paris, who lived five hours away. They arrived in early morning. Various other family members gathered throughout the night: Jerry's mother Reba, his sister Diane and her husband Bill, their daughters and sons-in-law. Art's foster mother and his foster sister, Fonda and Alice Hearst, appeared at dawn. I called our children, who also prepared to come.

We were truly an eclectic group as we huddled at the bedsides of Courtney and Zachary that night, joined in common concern and grief, but each with divided feelings and personal hells. A father, a daughter, a husband, a sister, and a mother were all in anguish.

It was an uneasy truce for all of us to be together. Art had been working for Jerry at the time of his and Courtney's divorce and ill feelings were still strong. Everyone was civil, probably due to the extreme shock. But the staff commented that they had never seen such a diverse family so cohesive. That cohesiveness was soon to dissolve.

CHAPTER TWO

ZACHARY LEAVES US

After a thorough family-doctor consultation early the second morning, we were told that there was no hope for Zachary's life. We were asked if we wanted to remove the life support systems. We all voiced our opinions, but the final decision had to be made by Art, who was not the custodial parent, but with Courtney near death, the logical one.

I'll never forget Art's whisper as he spoke more to himself than to anyone else, "I know what I must do, but I don't want to do it."

Unless you have been there, there is no way to share emotionally what having to make this decision meant. I knew the hurt in my heart, but could only imagine what Art and Christina were feeling. I could see the pain on the faces of the rest of the family. There seemed no other choice.

The machines came off. There were no indicators of life on Zachary's part. I believe that little Zachary died upon impact at the scene of the accident. This hard fact provided some comfort. The doctors had sustained him until Art could arrive. Zachary was and is his only biological son.

The doctor's words, "Zachary has gone home to Jesus," will always be with me and even today when I tell someone the number of our grandchildren, I may say, "One lives with Jesus."

The interdisciplinary team at the Children's Hospital had been phenomenally compassionate. The Lutheran chaplain found that Zachary had never been baptized and performed the sacrament at the bedside. This emotional moment will be remembered. A warm and concerned pediatrician spent the night with us at Zak's bedside. She never left once, which impressed me; I'm sure she had small children at home. The staff involved us in discussions, conferences, and decisions.

Medical and nursing professionals share an intimacy with families at life and death moments that no other professionals realize. Families are so vulnerable, which makes the health professionals carry a huge responsibility for their responses during these times. Warmth and sensitivity are needed; these we received.

Christina and her foster aunt, Alice, were led in art therapy or therapeutic drawing by the social worker. They were also taken to the chapel for a time of prayer and reflection, as well as writing a good-bye to Zachary in the chapel's registry. They both wrote that they were sorry they had been so mean to Zachary and sorry they had teased him so much. Sounded like the older sister of a pesky little brother.

Each of us was given a private time with Zachary at the end. I noted the usual cuts and scrapes on his strong little legs. He had few abrasions from the accident. No facial trauma. He looked absolutely normal. I recall his dark blonde hair with that strong cowlick on the right; he looked so peaceful, but so out of character of his usual "energizer-bunny" self. I, too, must have been in shock for I remember feeling numb as I sat there touching his little body. I kept thinking that tomorrow all of this will be over, and he'll come running in calling "Nanny, Nanny, Nanny," as he always did.

I had lost my parents, a beloved mother-in-law, a brother, the father of my children, and several friends, but nothing prepared me for the loss of this small child. The order was all wrong. Zak was my first grandson. I loved him so. He should have buried me. He did bury a part of me with him. A loss like this is not something that you ever get over; it's just something with which you learn to live.

I was happy when Art made the decision to donate Zachary's organs. Because of Zachary, five people have been given new leases on life. Many families are un-aware that they can give this gift of life, which can mean so much. There is no charge to the family. This decision can be made even prior to death with donor wallet cards available. We donated Zak's heart valves, kidneys and liver, and received an informational letter as to the recipients. The National Organ Donor Foundation may be contacted for more information. The web site infor-mation is listed in the Selected Resource section.

I have read that the spirit of a departed one can stay around for a few days to comfort loved ones. I wasn't sure I believed this, but in the first few days after Zachary's death, I felt his presence so close to me I felt I could touch him. I had never before experienced this. I could actually sense a presence very close to my back, almost like a soft weight on my shoulder and close to my ear. It was so healing.

Gradually, as I was a little stronger, the feeling of his presence faded, but I was already beginning to feel the comforting arms of God in even this small detail. It is true that He never leaves us (Matt. 28:20 NIV).

****

We left Courtney's bedside to return to Bloomington, Indiana, for Zachary's funeral. She was unaware that he had died. The funeral was sad for us, but we received the gift of warm and happy memories expressed by many people. The principal and teachers from Laurel Elementary School were there with poems and stories from Zak's kindergarten classmates. Even Penny, Zak's school bus driver, was there. Zak had always led me to believe Penny really disliked him and that she was a witch! Well, Penny was really a nice woman who said she secretly thought Zachary very cute but very mischievous.

So many friends, family members, and folks whom we hardly knew, came to share our sadness. Knowing that others were sharing our pain helped. Never underestimate your presence or words at these difficult times. Every word, every touch, every card, every visit gave us strength. A warm embrace meant so much.

Again I realized the importance of a funeral or at least a memorial service. With permission I quote Dr. Alan D. Wolfelt, who has done extensive work in the field of grieving.

> "More and more Americans are rejecting ritual when death occurs. Historically, funerals have provided a way of meeting social, psychological and spiritual needs during a time of transition. Among other functions, participation in ritual helps acknowledge the reality of the death, provides social support, assists in converting the relationship from presence to memory, and encourages the expression of a wide range of emotions. This growing rejection of ritual results in many bereaved people having complications in their mourning."

While my personal plans include only a memorial service, I am glad Zachary had a funeral. The word closure is inadequate at times like these, but Zak's funeral service helped me to let go of his temporal life here on earth.

At times during the funeral, we experienced real laughter. Laughter seems appropriate at funerals because we really are celebrating a life. Even in our sadness we celebrate a life that was with us for a time. During the viewing, there was a strong thunderstorm, and all lights went out. Candles were lit. This made things look eerie. At this point my dear friend and colleague, 80-year-old Dr. Richard Schell, who had delivered Zak's mother, said in his usual dry humor, "If I'd known the lights were going off, I wouldn't have worn a tie."

That levity softened the atmosphere. Thank you, Dr. Schell. Dr. Schell has since died.

Other memorable things helped ease the tension and our sadness. The fact that concert pianist John Schwandt of Saint Thomas Lutheran Church could offer an impromptu rendition of Zak's favorite song, "Dust in the Wind," added a poignant touch to the service. While sitting there, I couldn't help smiling as I recalled Zak's clear, sweet voice belting out this tune as he ran around the house.

Our pastors, Lowell Anderson and Walt Johnson, conducted the service and used some of my favorite scriptures from Lamentations 3 and Romans 8. Church member Carolyn Sowinski sang *Best du Beimir* in her beautiful soprano voice. As our daughter Julie said, it was a funeral fit for a king.

Our three-year-old granddaughter, Savannah, caught her mother Kathleen off guard when she said, "Mommy, why are you so sad? You'll see Zachary again."

How wise children are. They sometimes can see what we cannot see, and they certainly will go where we cannot go.

Nothing was more touching, though, than the little note that cousin Jimmy Helton had written during the service; he asked to put the note in the casket with Zak. I can't remember its exact contents, but it was written on a scrap of paper in that proud first- grade printing. That note accompanied Zak.

Such gestures left us with fond memories. To lose someone you love to death is sad, but happy memories are what sustain us. Down through the years, I have had to remember and focus on all the fun things with Zak. His life was short, but he left a legacy.

I've also had to realize that some lives are meant to be short on this earth. God knows all of the possible futures for all of us. I've come to accept Zachary's life of only six years.

For each family, Art had framed the imprint of Zachary's hands and feet along with an accompanying poem about memories. I do not know the author, but this hangs in my office. The poem is as follows:

> These are my little footprints; I made them just for you.
> Please know that they were done in love for all you do.
> Each time you see my footprints so neatly on the wall,
> fond memories will come back when I was with you all.
> These are my set of handprints; I made them just for you.
> Please know that they were done with love for all of you.

Each time you see my handprints so neatly on
the wall,
fond memories will come back when I was
with you all.

Zachary rests in Carmichael Cemetery in Greene
County, Indiana. It's a small graveyard in a lovely and
peaceful country setting. His grave is beside his pater-
nal grandmother, Lucille Harms. I've made a few trips
back, and Courtney feels she is near being ready to visit.

In memory of Zak, contributions from caring
individuals helped erect in the prayer garden of Saint
Thomas Lutheran Church what the children affection-
ately came to call "the Care Bear." It is a limestone bear,
sculptured by Morgan County artist Charles Schiefer.
As children and adults wander the garden, they are
drawn to touch the bear, and the bear becomes shinier
the more it is caressed. That little bear has already
spread joy. Even though we have moved from
Bloomington, it is good to know that something of

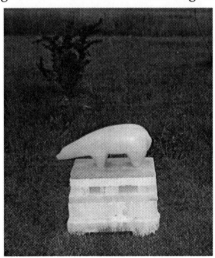

Zachary still re-
mains in the place
that meant so
much to us.

My grandson
Zachary still lives
in my heart and
always will. My
relationship with
him is just
changed, not gone.
It is no longer a
physical relation-
ship, but it is a

spiritual one. I still talk freely and openly to and about him. Often, only I know the catch in my throat when I explain that the little ceramic spirit house in my garden, right there beside my Saint Francis statue, represents Zachary to me. No, I don't believe Zak is really in that little house, but it's just a visual reminder to me that I know Zak's spirit is not gone, but endures.

Anne Jackson of Australia designs and makes the colored ceramic houses; she calls them spirit houses. She began making them after the death of her beloved husband, and the cottage industry has gotten away from her. I could not resist buying two to carry back on the plane. One was for Courtney. I keep mine where the elements, the wind, the rain, and the sun can flow through. Courtney keeps hers inside right beside her angel collection.

A few years after Zachary's death, I was in London, England, with a friend, Nancy Anderson. She picked up a card in a gift shop. While I'm not quite as pragmatic, its words speak my sentiments of continuing to hold a deceased loved one in your heart. The versing is as follows:

> DEATH is nothing at all. I have only slipped away into the next room. I am I, and you are you. Whatever we were to each other, that we still are. Call me by my old familiar name, speak to me in the easy way which you always used. Put no difference in your tone, wear no forced air of solemnity or sorrow. Laugh as we always laughed at the little jokes we enjoyed together. Play, smile, think of me, pray for me. Let my name be ever the household word that it always was, let it be spoken without effort, without the trace of a shadow on it. Life means all that it ever meant. It is the same as it ever was; there is unbroken continuity.

Why should I be out of mind because I am out of sight? I am waiting for you, for an interval, somewhere very near, just around the corner.

All is well.

Henry Scott Holland, 1847-1918,
Canon of St. Paul's Cathedral

I can't remember where I found the following verse, but it also expresses how we can experience a peace even about death if we feel God is near.

If Thou be near, go I with gladness to death and to eternal peace.

Ah, how content were thus my ending, if Thy dear hands were laid upon me, and gently closed my faithful eyes.

As I mentioned, I have lost several family members and friends to death. If I felt that death was the end, I would be devastated. Death doesn't have the final say. It has no sting for the believer, but represents the hope of a new life with God. This makes it bearable.

CHAPTER THREE

THE JOURNEY BEGINS

After the funeral, we began what some call "the vigilance" at Courtney's bedside. We wanted to be there all the times. She was still unconscious, being kept alive by a ventilator, a tracheotomy, and high-powered neurological medications. She knew nothing of our presence. Nothing could be done at this time for her many broken bones because of her coma. Had she been conscious, her pain would have been unbearable.

In the course of her hospitalization, she developed septicemia, pneumonia, a staphylococcus infection, respiratory alkalosis (an imbalance of gases), and thrombocytopenia (decreased platelets), presumably caused by one of the medications. The thrombocytopenia necessitated several blood and platelet transfusions. Much of this I did not know until after her discharge, for which I am thankful.

While we are indebted to the wonderful doctors, nurses, and others at University Hospital, we believe that only God gave Courtney back her life. Every time I would recount Courtney's massive injuries, I would stand in amazement. God had meant her to live. She had more than 31 different diagnoses or procedures during her hospitalization just at University Hospital.

We didn't know what to do but to wait, hope and pray. There is no such thing as anticipatory grief or any way in which we could have prepared ourselves to deal with this situation. There is no forewarning in sudden death, which seems to make its impact greater.

We were all in the initial stage of shock and knew we had to hold on to one another. We could not bear this grief alone. I have heard the stage of shock as compared to a padded wall, which softens the blow or the loss for a time at least. This is an appropriate analogy and is needed for most of us to be able to handle the initial phases of a tragedy.

Martha Hickman in her book titled *Healing After Loss* says this numbness is like a "benign form of anesthesia—giving our senses a time to rest before we reenter the whirlpool of torn lives, of shattered dreams, of anguished tears." She maintains this numbness is more than stoic acceptance of what is, but a "season" with its own logic, and one which will pass in time. I found these thoughts comforting.

I personally kept cascading between extremes of emotion. One minute I was in shock, and the next minute I was in denial with anger soon competing for position. I couldn't deny that Zak was dead and Courtney's critical condition, but I just couldn't sort out my emotions. I now realize that phases of sorrow have no fences around them, but that slipping from one to the other or even sliding backward is what we do. Something within us makes us take as long as we need within these boundaries of grief.

Jerry, Christina, Courtney's sister, her brother and his family, and Conrad and I spent long days and nights at Courtney's bedside. We gave support to one another, which is all that can be done in the acute phase of a tragedy.

Our other children and their families traveled long distances to see Courtney. We couldn't have felt more love from our children at this time. They kept us going as well as made us feel proud for how each of them rose to the occasion.

Our pastors, our extended family, and many caring friends came to offer comfort. Friends in Cincinnati, Pam and Pete Gillon, opened their home to us as a resting place. The hospital also had a respite hotel room for families. We were on the receiving end of much love. It felt so good and so right. It helped us remain strong. I remember this now when I am on the giving end.

I didn't know until much later that my friend's son, Dr. Nathan Millikan, a resident at University Hospital, had been slipping in daily to check on Courtney and, no doubt, to whisper a prayer. Thank you, Nathan. How good it was to know your trained eye looked on her daily. Nathan and Courtney had been children together.

Courtney was on many prayer chains, even one on the Internet. Prayer was our powerful link to peace. As grieved as I was, I did feel the peace of God. I knew this had to be supernatural. God's promise of peace "not as the world gives" was so real to me those days (John 14:27 NIV). It was enough to sustain me.

Saint Paul's words from Romans 5 (NIV) were also encouraging: "...we know that suffering produces endurance, and endurance produces character, and character produces hope, and hope does not disappoint us, because God's love has been poured into our hearts through the Holy Spirit that has been given to us."

Blanket acceptance of these promises was not without initial struggle, but as I learned to rest in God, they became my comfort. Many times I told God I was tired of having my character built or being refined like gold. I told Him that I would be happy to settle for being bronze for awhile, but these promises became and still are my articles of faith.

Each of us began to mourn in our individual ways. Mourning is simply the outward expression of our inner grief. I know that at first I was not able to talk about the accident. It was so painful, and I felt so exposed to the world. Tears were always close to the surface and at times overflowing. I learned though that each time I was able to talk about the loss of Zachary, I was able to let go of his death a little more. I have also learned that the tears of grief have been scientifically analyzed, as compared with tears of joy, and those tears of grief contain toxins. How beautiful to think of our tears of grief as purifying.

I knew my heartache for Courtney's condition was only beginning.

Courtney's siblings, Julie Martin Federico and Michael Martin, had hearts so filled with pain. They had barely gotten over their father's death of just a few years earlier. But they were there for Courtney at every opportunity, even when she did not know they were there. They were her best cheering section and injected humor at every opportunity. They came to spend that first Thanksgiving with Courtney at the hospital while Conrad and I took a needed break. We made the already planned trip to California for the holiday with some of our other children.

Julie's suffering has taken a long time to heal. She and Courtney were close. I have yet to lose a sister, so I can't identify with what Julie knew was a distinct possibility. She made many trips from Denver just to be there even though Courtney never knew. Julie, as counselor, brought the gift of emotional intelligence to the whole tragedy. We all benefited from her wisdom.

Men seem to grieve differently than women. My husband, Conrad, has a very pragmatic view of death and simply sees death as just a transition. While he may feel sad, that is not his prevailing emotion. He says death really tests your belief in a hereafter. Conrad has lost a dear brother unexpectedly and recently both parents, so he speaks from his experience. He is right as far as how he views death and grief, but I must go through the emotions in my own way. I must visit the pain; this is how I am healed.

The words of Shakespeare come to mind when thinking of how Conrad deals with grief. "Give sorrow words; the grief that does not speak whispers the oe'r fraught heart and bids it break." Telling and retelling our story helps establish the reality of the event. I am thankful for dear sisters, friends, and other dear family members who listened to me again and again. This is how I am helped, but we all grieve in our individual ways.

Many people never complete their grieving. Unfortunately they allow it to affect them for the rest of their lives in an adverse way. With time and help, I found it was possible to get beyond the loss.

Jerry, whose whole pattern of life had evaporated, had to rebuild again. He turned to his work, which is what men often do. Work gave him a focus. He says he has learned a new appreciation of the gift of each day, particularly each day that he and Courtney have together.

****

At week's end, we began to wonder if Courtney would ever come back to us. There did not seem to be any progress. Jerry was feeling a lot of pressure to make the right decisions regarding Courtney. Given her seemingly hopeless situation, we discussed whether the ventilator should just be turned off, but a wise neurosurgeon cautioned that it was far too early to make such a drastic decision. We were all anxious about the quality of life Courtney would have if she did come back, while simultaneously anxious that she might not come back.

Courtney was only 32 years old and had made no living will. I had seen many patients in Courtney's condition and knew exactly what her life could be. Is one ever too young to make a living will? If Courtney had had a living will requesting no extraordinary interventions should she be critically ill, and if we had taken her off life support, we would never have seen her miraculous recovery. I have no perfect answer for families. Every family must arrive at its own decisions, but this whole area of end-of-life decisions for the young is perhaps one needing more attention.

None of us can know what we would do unless we have been there, and no one can make the decision for us. I know how agonizing it was for Art to make the decision regarding Zachary. I could see the same anguish in Jerry's eyes and could feel it in my own soul as well.

During these days, we each did a lot of soul searching. We unconsciously played the "what if game." What would we do if Courtney returned in a vegetative state? What would we do if she didn't make it at all? How would we handle any of this? How would we feel? I didn't think I could stand the pain of her being in a vegetative state, but I realized that many families have had to bear having a loved one in a chronic vegetative state. I immediately thought of the recent Terry Shivo case. Somehow I knew I would be given strength as I needed it.

I had to wrestle long and hard with the fact that my daughter had alcohol and marijuana in her bloodstream at the time of the accident. Her alcohol level was not above the legal limit and there was only a trace of marijuana, which I'm told could have been weeks old, but they were there nonetheless. This knowledge was as if a sledgehammer had pounded me. I was in disbelief for days and couldn't allow myself to dwell on the fact. I had a hard time discussing it. I felt a gamut of emotions from anger to the worst sadness I have known. With Courtney comatose, I thought I will never know the real story.

Did she get distracted by Zak, look back and take her eyes off the road? This likely happened for they used to play the game called "Quiet like a Mouse" when they were in the car. The purpose of the game was to keep the child quiet while riding. Zak would zip up his lips and pretend to be quiet like a mouse. The first one to laugh or talk lost the game. I can just see Courtney looking back at Zachary and laughing. I had to believe it was an accident, and over time this is exactly what I have come to believe: it was an accident. A dreadful accident.

There is no way I feel that God ordained Zachary to die that day or Courtney to have such severe injuries. I simply do not believe it was God's will for them to be so injured. This is not how God works. God's nature is to desire good for us. In our humanness we can make ill-fated decisions, which can adversely affect our lives.

I have learned that with life comes times of sadness. It doesn't mean that God has left us. It means we are human. Rabbi Krushner was right when he wrote "bad things can happen to good people." It's what we do with the bad things that tell the real story. We can move forward into hope or backward into chronic grief. It's a painful, difficult choice, and sometimes our choices are indeed imperfect.

I did find God's sweet, supernatural peace, which was waiting there for me all the time. But I can easily understand why some people succumb to alcohol, drugs, or other ill-coping behaviors to numb their pain. I, too, wanted to be numbed and relieved of the pain. I was made fully aware of my human limitations.

A close Christian friend who has had many illnesses said, "I don't know why God has spoken to me so often through illnesses." Like Barbara, I don't know why this tragedy took place, but God walked with me down this pathway. I can only continue to believe and hold on as Barbara has done throughout her life. Brucie is another dear friend who has endured many medical problems in her life, but she has a faith that is inspiring to me. God does help us in our infirmities, but it's good to have real-life examples like Barbara and Brucie for inspiration.

When we said good night to Courtney, we left Mozart and Beethoven tapes playing. Courtney had always enjoyed classical music, and we were hopeful it might help her regain consciousness. We had heard of the man who had awakened from a long coma while Tchaikovsky's "1812 Overture" was playing. We were doing what we thought might be helpful.

We weren't aware then, but we were using medical music therapy. Most of us have known intuitively that music is therapeutic, but using music for medical therapy is becoming increasingly popular. It's now felt that music can be an audio analgesic or audio sedative, which can affect the patient's biomedical or psycho social state. Simply said: music is good for the soul.

Tami Briggs is a harpist who goes into hospital settings and plays for patients. She firmly believes in the therapeutic benefits of music; it is her ministry. I have seen and heard Tami. I have her CD called "Love's Journey" and can attest to the calming serenity of her music. Her web site is listed in the Selected Resources at the end of the book.

I am also reminded of the Bible story of how the disturbed King Saul ordered the shepherd boy David to play the harp to soothe his troubled soul (I Samuel 16:27 NIV). Even long ago the calming effects of music were known.

At a recent conference I picked up a flyer that listed other benefits of music therapy: to mask ambient noise; to serve as a focus of attention; to reinforce learning; to promote stress reduction; to aid in pain management; to help in addictions recovery; to calm the elderly, and to increase workplace effectiveness.

I'm confident that music will take its place among medical therapies. To me, there is no doubt that music is a wonderful gift to us and has many roles in our lives. Nothing is as soothing or as freeing to the soul as music. Its energy is an impetus that moves us to action. Art also works in many of the same ways.

At the time of the accident, Courtney's sister Julie was a middle school counselor in Evergreen, Colorado, and the art students there sent fantastic acrylic chalk drawings, which we hung around Courtney's bed. They were all wonderful, but three in particular stood out to me, and I have them to this day. One says "For those who dream there is no such word as impossible." Another says, "The grand essentials of happiness are: something to do, something to love and something to hope for (Chalmers)." The third one says, "The best memories are of the good times, may every minute be

the best memorie"-(spelled this way). These simple
drawings calmed us, renewed us and encouraged us.
The kids gave of themselves without knowing the
powerful impact of the drawings.

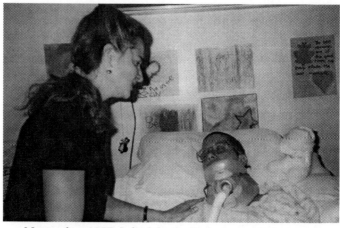

November 1997: Julie Martin Federico and Courtney

Music and art. What would life be without these?
Picasso says "Art washes away from the soul the dust of
everyday life." We were hoping it would wash away the
cobwebs of coma.

****

On day eleven, Courtney opened her eyes. Michael
was the first to see her open her eyes. We were all very
excited, but that excitement soon dimmed when we saw
the vacant look behind her pretty blue eyes. Where was
our Courtney? These were not her eyes. Hope waned
again.

We each did that which we thought might help.
Jerry would whisper lovingly into her ear and the rest of
us talked and read to her, but mainly we just kept
hoping and praying. Christina was always close beside

her mother, often with her head upon Courtney's pillow. Christina seemed so comfortable with her mother. She didn't seem anxious. I wondered if she really understood the gravity of her mother's condition. Like any twelve year old, she probably thought her mother was just very sick, but that she would get better and leave the hospital. Christina either couldn't or wouldn't talk about her feelings or worries. We didn't pry either. We waited, each in our own world of emotion.

After several days, Courtney's eyes became brighter, and she was able to respond to simple commands. Hope began to return. She was moved from the surgery intensive care unit to an orthopedic unit. She had surgery on her left leg and a feeding tube placed. We think she recognized us, but that is about all. She was unable to speak. We talked to her as if she could understand. In truth, I don't think anything was registering with her at this time. She had no idea of where she was or what had happened. Jerry finally helped her understand that she had been in an accident. She remembered nothing about the accident. In fact, she remembered little at all.

We did not speak of Zachary to her.

So began the long journey.

CHAPTER FOUR

CHRISTINA NEEDS AN ANCHOR

With Courtney hospitalized indefinitely and Jerry on leave from work to be at her side, what was to happen to Christina? Who would care for her? What about school? She had already been out two weeks. With so much turmoil, Christina's welfare had taken a back seat; her well being now surfaced to high priority. Christina made us realize this as she kept repeating the question, "Where am I going to live?"

One can only guess just what was going on in her twelve-year-old mind, as she did not open up or show much emotion during this time. I've no doubt she felt deep emotion, but Christina had always been very private about her feelings. How much should a child have to bear? I was again thankful that the hospital social worker had done so much emotional therapy with her. I remember thinking God gives needed resiliency to children. Thank you, God.

Conrad and I wanted Christina to live with us, but knew our household and lifestyle were no longer geared toward children. Uncle Michael and Aunt Stephanie were very willing to have Christina, but they lived a thousand miles away and Christina's seeing Courtney, Jerry, and Art would have been difficult. None of us could live with Christina in her home so that she would not have had to be uprooted. There was no perfect answer.

Art adamantly expressed his wish to have Christina live with his family. I turned this over in my mind many ways. Did she represent his last link to his son Zachary? His only blood connection. I now know that Art was doing what he thought best for Christina.

Relations between the Larson family and the Paris family had been strained even before the accident, so when Art wanted Christina to live with them, the idea was unsettling to me. As her legal father, he had the most legitimate right even if he was not the custodial parent. We were told that we would probably lose if we petitioned for her. Art filed for temporary custody; we filed for grandparents' rights, and Christina moved five hours north to Griffith, Indiana, to a new life.

Watching my young granddaughter move away was difficult. I felt that I had lost Zachary, maybe Courtney, and now I was losing Christina. I felt protective and did not want her that far away without mother, grandmother, or blood relation in a family that I hardly knew. I was very uncomfortable but was again made aware of my lack of legal rights in the whole situation. This was not an easy period.

In spite of my lawyer's counsel that I would lose in a custody claim, my children felt that I should have fought harder to keep Christina. I reluctantly accepted her move, because I did not want to cause more chaos in her young life. I had to have faith at this point, because I could not see ahead, and specters of concern loomed. As years have passed, my faith has been rewarded.

Art and his wife, Dawn, welcomed Christina and did their best to provide the needed emotional support. They arranged counseling for Christina and, in time, she did discuss her feelings with her counselor.

Paris' had a family rule: at least one hour every evening Christina had to be sociable and had to be out of her room with the rest of the family. This rule stemmed from the fact that at home Christina had preferred to stay in her room most of the time.

Christina's new family included 13-year-old step-sister Krysten, 14-year-old stepbrother Brandon, and three year old stepsister Ashlynn. Sasha, the cat, and Max, the dog, completed the family. Dawn also had parents, siblings and extended family in town, so large loving groups welcomed Christina. They readily incorporated her into the family circle.

I think that finding an active family environment was healing for Christina. Her usual family life was gone. Her little brother was dead, her mother was in a coma, and her stepfather was nearly overcome with grief. Where was her anchor? What depths of anguish does a twelve year old feel when told to handle such grief? I feel that God gave Christina the same peace and comfort that He gave to me. But as she matures, she'll have to revisit her feelings. I pray for her complete recovery from grief at that time.

The routine of family life with parents, sisters, a brother, and pets helped restore normalcy to the turmoil she must have felt. She began a new school, but Krysten and Brandon were there to smooth the rough spots. A few friends multiplied, a church home was found, and her room soon looked as if she had been a lifelong occupant. My concerns began to lessen. When Christina added a parakeet named Blue and an albino snake named Malachi, I felt she was home.

* * * *

Christina saw her mother at every opportunity, which, in those early days of Courtney's hospitalization, was about every other weekend for month after month. Conrad and I took on the responsibility for facilitating these trips, since the Paris and Larson families were still estranged. These long road trips were a lot to ask of Christina, but she wanted to come. I feel that Courtney was aware that she was there even though they could not communicate. In the early weeks after the accident, Christina would simply lie back on the pillow beside Courtney with their heads very close. If it was emotionally upsetting for Christina to see her mother like this, she never let it be known.

When I looked at them together, role reversal was what came to my mind. It was like Christina, the mother, was offering comfort to Courtney, the child.

These trips between Bloomington and Griffith with a pick-up point at the Cracker Barrel in Lafayette, Indiana, proved a disguised blessing. Christina learned a lot about us, and we learned much more about this quiet twelve year old. We listened to her music, she listened to our stories, and even the silence became comfortable.

Sometimes Christina did homework during these long drives; sometimes she slept. Occasionally both Conrad and I went to pick her up; but usually only one of us went. I won't deny the frequent travel was a strain, but because of the trips, Christina and Conrad developed a close relationship, which they may not have had otherwise.

Again, we were realizing that positive things were happening from this terrible experience. Maybe it was because I had quit asking, "Why God?" and simply had begun to say, "I accept." This is a hard lesson to learn when you hurt so much.

Looking back, I realize that life could have gone a number of directions for Christina. She could have become rebellious and joined a wrong crowd. She could have tried drugs to numb her pain, or she could have become emotionally disabled. But she did none of these. I'm sure the pain was and is there, but with the help of God, friends, and family she made a new life. She became very active in her church, the Griffith Christian Church, finding strength and comfort.

She graduated from high school and had a wonderful celebration. I laughed and said to her, "Girl, you have a car, a job, a cell phone, a credit card, go to college, and have a boyfriend. What more do you want?" She just smiled.

Christina still does not say much about Zachary, but I know she remembers. I dislike tattoos, but I became emotional when Christina showed me her tattoo of a little angel carrying a banner with Zak written on it. Courtney, Jerry, and Christina all have the same tattoo. It's their way of remembering.

Art, Dawn, Courtney, and Jerry have continued to provide consistent and firm love for Christina. This love will continue to guide the rest of her life.

It is good to see that much is being written about children and grief and for children who have lost a loved one to death. Children need every bit as much help as an adult, if not more, when facing such a crisis. All of us are usually ill prepared to deal with loss. All of us need to make a choice to reconcile or resolve the grief, but generally we need help finding the way.

CHAPTER FIVE

REALITY MUST BE FACED

After four weeks in the hospital, Courtney went to a nursing home called Lincoln Center in Connersville, Indiana. This was close to their home. The bittersweet irony is that Courtney and Jerry had actually been married at Lincoln Center, because this was the only way that Jerry's mother Reba, a patient there at the time, could attend the wedding.

Courtney went to Lincoln Center because she wasn't strong enough for physical rehabilitation. She was still unable to communicate. When strong enough, she would be moved to Hook's Rehabilitation Center in Indianapolis, Indiana.

The Hook's personnel knew how anxious we were to get rehabilitation started and accepted Courtney just one week after she went to Lincoln Center. They also knew that for us to have our young Courtney in a nursing home environment was almost more than we could bear. Their acceptance was too early, for within seven days she was back at Lincoln Center. She could not stand upright for the length of time needed to initiate physical therapy.

The Lincoln period was very difficult for everyone. We had not been able to grieve for Zachary because we were so concerned about Courtney. Events seemed overwhelming to us. We were short with one another. I felt that a nursing home was not the place for Courtney. Courtney's needs were so different than the other residents. Deep down, I was afraid this would be where she would remain. There were misunderstandings with the staff. Jerry was so grieved and so stressed that he was not at his best. This was one of our darkest periods.

Someone stayed with Courtney most of the time because, although awake, she still had coma behavior. It was explained that Courtney would not remember any of this time, and she does not. Her behavior was very uninhibited, which was expected from the brain injury. While her behavior was sometimes funny, this meant she had to have constant surveillance.

One night when alone, she climbed out of bed in spite of the heavy cast on her left leg. Her frail roommate said felt she had to watch Courtney. She told us that she had stayed awake much of the night guarding Courtney. We then had safety concerns.

Courtney became the topic of interest for other Lincoln patients who could be mobile. One afternoon, a sweet little lady navigated her wheelchair in and said, "I just want to see this Courtney that everyone is talking about. What happened to you, Honey?"

In true uninhibited coma behavior, Courtney answered her, "I———up."

The little lady gasped, "Oh!" and wheeled from the room. I was both amused and shocked. This response was definitely not Courtney but did show how affected her brain had been. All of this type of behavior eventually faded, and she remembers none of it.

Jerry went back to work but spent nights sleeping at her bedside. I took leave from work and stayed during the day. The staff did look after Courtney and the fact that Jerry's sister Diane worked there helped us feel a little more secure. We each tried to take care of ourselves, to get rest, but I'll confess it was near impossible and fatigue was ever lurking.

I'll always remember that it was at Lincoln Center that speech therapy was started. I'll never forget Courtney's call to me the day her tracheotomy was removed.

A soft, raspy voice whispered, "Mom, I love you."

Never have I heard dearer words, even if they were husky and hard to understand. How wonderful that she could talk!

After three, long weeks at Lincoln Center, she was again transferred to Hook's and was able to stay this time. We were elated and felt that perhaps our Courtney would return to us after all. Hook's Rehabilitation is connected with Community Hospital in Indianapolis. They have an excellent rehabilitation program. Courtney was placed on a head trauma unit.

* * * *

At this eight-week mark, we thought Courtney understood that she had been in an accident. She understood that Zachary was dead only because Jerry had finally been able to tell her, and she seemed to blindly accept without emotion. We had been apprehensive to tell her about Zachary for fear she would sink into a depression, but in reality Courtney was not at the point of real understanding. She talked to us, she looked at us, but she was not there.

In those early stages of recovery, I believe our heavenly Father was protecting her from feeling or remembering too much, because He knew she would not be able to handle the anguish. It turned out she had no memory of Zak, no memory of the accident or of events two or three years prior to the accident.

When she was sufficiently recovered and much stronger, some of this memory came back, but that took years. In the early days, she acknowledged Jerry, Christina, me, and others, but she couldn't with any detail remember Zak. My worry about her emotional state when she found out about Zachary's death had been needless. Her lack of memory and a design far greater than mine had intervened.

Courtney's traumatic brain injury involved several areas of her brain. She had a fracture with bruising in the back and left side of her skull. She had hemorrhages on both sides of the brain tissue. There was a question of whether her left internal carotid artery at the base of the skull was dissected, but it was not. Truth is, her brain had taken a severe beating in the accident. While her whole brain was affected, the left side suffered the most. Speech ability lies on the left side of the brain.

Many emotions are also centered on the left side of the brain. Her affect was flat and blunted for a long time. She was unable to shed tears because she couldn't feel emotion. This unemotional behavior of my daughter was hard for me to understand at first. I just kept thinking she would show some emotion about something, but she didn't. It took a long time.

Years later when she could feel emotions, she joked, "I liked it better when I couldn't feel so much!"

At Hook's, Courtney had a daily program designed to stretch her abilities. Her schedule was taped to the arm of her wheelchair so that she could see what activity came next. She went to speech therapy, occupational therapy, cognitive therapy, and physical therapy.

The therapy Courtney liked best was the pet therapy program in which owners brought their pets to the bedside. I thought she was hallucinating when she told me she had petted a cat. Courtney has always had a kitten in her life, sometimes two. Christina shares the same love. Courtney's Aunt Betty shares this deep love for cats, too.

I was amused when she said she had received communion twice one Sunday. She could not make the Catholic priest understand that she had already taken communion from the Lutheran chaplain earlier.

Wisely, she said, "I didn't think it would hurt." I didn't either.

Courtney had to relearn the basic rudimentary life skills, even bladder training. She had to learn to talk, to write, to crawl, and to walk again. Her ability to read was intact but with little comprehension or concentration.

Relearning basic life skills was not easy. From my observations, it seemed much harder the second time around. The staff had her on a two-hour bladder retraining schedule, and it was so hard to tell her she could not go to the bathroom any more often. In her compulsiveness, she was asking to go every ten to fifteen minutes. The task of getting her to the toilet was not a simple feat either. She had a heavy leg cast, was wheelchair bound, and had no muscle strength of her own.

We were so glad she finally was in therapy but found it painful to watch her try to accomplish the most basic things. Even swallowing was problematic; fluids had to be thickened so that they were not aspirated into the lungs. I watched and recalled a little baby learning these same things years ago.

Talking was tiring for Courtney, but listening to her took energy and patience as well. I often wanted to finish sentences for her. My energy, though, was minuscule compared to her efforts. She worked to create her words. Her brain simply was not making the right synapses. Sometimes even today she waits for her brain to catch up with her words.

She had wonderful physical therapists at Hook's, but her struggle at the parallel bars was the hardest for me to watch. I remembered her first steps at eight months old. Now I held my breath as I watched her painful efforts to put one foot in front of the other. The walking was the last skill for her to reacquire, because the bones in her left leg were not healing properly, and she could not bear weight for quite awhile.

She returned to surgery a second time for this leg, which further delayed her walking. Today she is challenged with almost constant arthritic pain in the left leg because of the breaks.

Her voice accent, once she came out of the coma, was English sounding. Was this DNA from the past talking? I was "Mother!" which she pronounced very distinctively and drawn out. Christina was "Daughter!" which was crisply enunciated. Her neurologist said it was not unusual for a coma patient to speak with a different accent when awakened. He related the story of a New York African American who spoke with an unmistakable Jamaican accent after his coma.

Eventually, Courtney returned to her usual speaking pattern, but to this day enunciates words more precisely than before. She said regaining speech has been particularly hard, because she thinks more slowly than she can talk. The initial effort was very physically tiring for her.

Courtney spent almost three months in rehab, but she remembers little. She was with us, she talked to us, but she was really somewhere else in her mind. The hospital was over an hour from both Jerry and us, but we made the trip often. All of Christina's visits were spent at the hospital.

As she neared release, she was allowed brief home visits. I'll never forget using the slide board to transfer her from wheelchair to car and my worry of having her fall. We also had to have a neighbor help us lift her wheelchair up our steps as we had no handicap ramp.

But Courtney was making progress, and we were glad. We, in fact, were witnessing a miracle.

I would look at Courtney and think "I can't believe you are able to do what you are doing." Medical reason said she should have been dead or at least a vegetable. Courtney said that the things that kept her going were Jerry and Christina and thinking of Zachary as an angel in heaven. These were her small threads of hope.

It's very comforting to think of a child who has died as a little angel in heaven. While it's true, according to the Bible, that angels carried Zachary safely to the arms of Jesus (Luke 16: 23 NIV), human beings do not become angels. Angels and humans are separate entities. People are born and angels are created. Angels were created by God out of nothing before the creation of the world and carry out many functions for God.

We're given to saying, "You're an angel" when referring to someone, but humans are humans and angels are angels. Today's emphasis on angels, or angelology as it's called, has proliferated almost beyond belief. There are angel stores, angel books, angel figurines, angel wallpapers, angel societies, and, of course, angel stories. People want to believe in angels. Belief in angels brings comfort and hope to many of us.

I am persuaded that during this time I encountered two different angels who were sent to strengthen and encourage me. In one incident, I had just taken our daughter Julie Martin Federico to the Indianapolis Airport for her return flight to Denver. All our children made so many sacrifices to come during this time. We know it was not easy for them. Their efforts meant so much; only a parent can know what the presence of children means during a tragedy. Trips to the airport were a frequent occurrence.

On this particular trip, I was weary and recalled that I still had another two and half hour drive ahead of me back to the Cincinnati Hospital. A feeling of heaviness settled upon me as I slumped on the telephone stool and started to call Conrad.

Before dialing, I looked out to the corridor and found this tall, slim man making direct eye contact with me. He smiled and I thought, "Well, he must know me."

He looked familiar, but I couldn't place him. To this day I can describe everything about him. He had brown eyes, dark brown, curly hair, and was quite handsome. He wore a dark suit, a white shirt, and carried an overcoat and umbrella, not your average dressed airline passenger these days. His face resembled my brothers' faces when they were young.

He kept looking directly at me, kept smiling, and began to nod his head as if to say, "It's going to be okay." He just kept on walking and maintaining eye contact with me for what seemed a long time before he was lost in the crowd. Immediately, I sensed in my heart that this was an angel. I certainly had not been thinking about angels at that time but knew without question the identity of this person. An unusual feeling of serene peace engulfed me. I sat for several minutes, calmed and strengthened. I have never felt such renewal.

I feel we do not give enough credit to angels, who are spiritual beings assigned particular tasks for God. I believe that angels are constantly around us. They carry out many functions, such as helping, protecting, intervening, guiding, and doing battle for God. They can bring messages, they surround us at death, or they may just comfort and strengthen us. Many people can share wonderful angel stories.

On one other previous occasion, I had stumbled as I was walking and knew with certainty that I would fall face first on the concrete.

Thoughts of "Oh, no, I can't fall. I need to work and have so much to do," flashed across my mind.

I hadn't meant it as a prayer for it all happened so fast, but God must have heard it as one. Instantly, I felt a soft wind beneath my body, which lifted me just enough for me to regain my footing, and I did not fall. I could hardly believe what happened. I have no doubt this was a protecting angel.

I had one other angel episode while Courtney was in the surgery intensive care unit. Again, this was an encouraging angel. My friend Betsy Bosin had driven with me to the hospital that day, and we were just leaving Courtney's room. Betsy had said that never in her life had she seen such an ill person. As we walked out, a female chaplain carrying a meal tray was entering. In the two weeks we had been there, I had not seen one meal tray arrive, much less carried by a chaplain. People on ventilators don't eat meals. I thought how strange to see a meal tray arriving.

To my surprise she asked me, "Who are you here for?"

She looked me directly in the eye when she asked the question.

As soon as I answered "Courtney Larson," she began nodding her head in just the same fashion as the other angel had done. She didn't say another word—just continued carrying the tray forward.

Something felt familiar, and again I was flooded with a serene sense of comfort and peace. I whispered to Betsy, "She's an angel."

I can to this day also describe every detail of this woman. She wore a white clerical collar and a light blue, two-piece pique suit. She was shorter than average and somewhat stocky. Her hair was reddish, her eyes dark, her skin the color of a latte coffee, and she had freckles across the bridge of her nose; a strong, compassionate looking woman.

These episodes I have kept in my heart and shared discriminately, but I have no doubt about them. God does meet us in our need. Whether these were just coincidental human beings, which I doubt, who crossed my path or whether they were heavenly angels is not as important as knowing that God in His providence knew and cared for my being at this time.

One of my favorite Bible passages is Psalms 91:11-12 NIV: "For He will command His angels concerning you to guard you in all your ways; they will lift you up in their hands, so that you will not strike your foot against a stone."

I take this verse to mean that we each have our own guardian angel whose job it is to watch after us. This may be an inconceivable idea to many, but I suggest giving it thought. I am enamored with the idea of a spiritual bodyguard.

Down through the years, I had appropriated this particular verse from Psalms for Christina and Zachary and had given names to their guardian angels. Christina's angel is named Irma and Zak's was Fred. I had many conversations with Irma and Fred; I still talk on a regular basis to Irma. Fred has a new assignment now.

I can imagine the angels as they go over their daily assignments. I hope they have a sense of humor about being assigned to those of us having less than a sunny day. Give your Guardian Angel a reason to smile today. You might be surprised!

CHAPTER SIX

In for the Long Haul

On January 28, 1998, almost four months after the accident, Courtney had recovered enough to be released from the hospital. She wasn't well by any means, but the caretaking responsibility was now Jerry's, her husband.

During this whole journey, my family and I had to realize that even though we cared so much, we did not have the legal right or responsibility regarding medical decisions about Courtney's care. We were not privy to a lot of the medical information. A few times this brought discord between Jerry and ourselves, but we had to learn to give up any right we may have felt to influence the circumstances. We did manage to work together, but I won't say it was easy. To be a mother and not be able to influence medical decisions about your comatose daughter is hard.

Jerry has been right by Courtney's side since the night of the accident and still is today. Jerry is a very private person, but he certainly showed his love for Courtney. His whole life was changed at once. His stepson was gone. His stepdaughter moved, and his wife was at death's door. He had many low days, but he managed to keep going.

He immersed himself in his work, which has brought him a great deal of satisfaction in terms of projects he and others have been able to achieve for the company and the community. One project is a model center in Connersville, Indiana, for lifelong learning for all ages. The center is called the Community Education Coalition.

Jerry has remained Courtney's strongest supporter. He encouraged Courtney to return to physical therapy when it became obvious she needed more improvement in her walking. He's made time for numerous medical visits for Courtney and has tried to help her maximize her potential. He's applauded her keeping her own checkbook, encouraged her in use of the computer and has been tolerant of her slow, but steady progress in all areas of daily living. He has believed in her, is there for her low days, and has also been a big part of the miracle of her life.

Since Courtney could not be left alone at first, she and Jerry stayed two months at the house of Diane and Bill Hensley, Jerry's sister and brother-in-law. Courtney remembers how Bill helped her memory by telling her the dinner menu and later quizzing her about it. Until she was able to give her own heparin shots, Bill was the shot giver since he gave himself daily insulin shots. Living in someone else's home required patience and understanding all around, but this arrangement did allow Jerry to work and allow Courtney to be with someone.

At last she was able to be left alone during the day, and they were able to return home. What a happy day! At first, Jerry did all the cooking and housework. Courtney's short-term memory was very poor at this point. She was afraid to use the stove for fear she would leave on the burners. She didn't complain but said fried eggs for dinner became monotonous. She made cold cuts for lunch and in time felt she could manage the microwave. Very low stamina and physical instability prevented her doing housework. These were really hard days, but we were all so thankful Courtney was with us that any hardship seemed easy.

To cope with a fragile emotional state in these early stages of recovery, Courtney placed photos of tranquil scenery around the house. She said such pictures were soothing. She had meditation spots such as her rocker beside the aquarium. She listened to music, tried to exercise, and read. She sat in the sun whenever possible. She had few visitors, because a lot of activity caused her to feel confused and agitated.

Jerry and Courtney live in the country with woodland views from their windows. Country living and nature have always been close to Courtney's heart, and during her recovery she said that the woods with all the birds and animals were very tranquilizing. Many of us seek solace in nature; I know that I do. Its silence restores our souls and instills a sense of hope.

Riding in a car was very traumatic for Courtney at first. She felt very anxious. She tried listening to tapes with earphones or concentrating on a pictorial focal point. A two-hour trip to my house was almost more than she could manage. It took about one year for her to be able to tolerate riding without excessive anxiety. Riding still keeps her tense, but she has made great strides.

Courtney, by medical standards, should have died with Zachary. She certainly shouldn't have recovered as well. We were told that whatever progress she had made at eighteen months would be her performance level. Medical predictions can miss the mark. We were most grateful for this fact. Courtney continued to gain after the eighteen-month mark; even today will surprise us with something she says or does. It was only with God's daily help that we were able to keep hope alive.

I don't mean to say Courtney has regained all her previous capacities. Not by any means, but she continues making progress and regaining control of her life. She is alive today, but she is very aware there is a special reason. A second chance has been given to our daughter. She's doing her best to take advantage of the privilege.

The head injury left her a completely different personality. The old Courtney is gone. We have had a new daughter to learn to know and love. We laugh at the differences as she will later relate. Cognitively, all the previous skills are not there, yet her present ability to be analytical and to problem solve is amazing. She's learning to compensate for her new compulsions, which she will tell you about. Decreased physical abilities have caused her to develop creatively in other areas such as cooking, gardening, jewelry making, and a correspondence ministry.

As a young person, Courtney had been very casual about neatness, particularly regarding her room. I remember collecting food, dishes, and other discarded items from her room, from under her bed, and from her closet. Clothes were in heaps everywhere. She was comfortable and none of this bothered her. Now it is a different story.

She says that when asked where something was, she used to say, "Oh, in the house."

But now she says, "I can tell you, it's in the house, in the bedroom, in the chest, second drawer on the right side."

And, indeed, everything in her house has a place. When she takes off a pair of shoes, she lines them up in her closet. On one occasion, I persuaded her to leave her house shoes in the living room. She did, but first thing in the morning, they were lined up in the closet. This is not the Courtney I once knew!

I've noticed that this Courtney doesn't mind telling her opinion on a subject, while the old Courtney offered few opinions even if she had them. Now she knows what she wants and what she doesn't want. She is refreshingly candid. She and Conrad enjoy bantering back and forth. When she likes or wants something, she lets you know in such an endearing way that you just want to give it to her.

She seems very aware of people's feelings and has an increased sensitivity about her, which she did not have before. She is very quick to offer thanks and to praise people; the thanks which I receive for doing something for her are sweet and warm to my heart.

The new Courtney is tougher. She has more patience, strength, and perseverance. I find this phenomenal because, God knows, she needs these character traits now.

After almost two years, Courtney finally recovered enough to know that her little son had died in the accident. Initially, she mercifully remembered nothing of the accident and accepted that Zachary had died, but only because she had been told.

There's much about him that she cannot remember, but bits and pieces of memory seem to be returning. I wonder if in time her mind may be healed enough to remember more, but she may never regain complete understanding. She remembers little of childhood friends, prior events, or her deceased father.

It has been perplexing as well as fascinating to see what she remembers and what she doesn't. She is a good example, though, that the brain's pathways indeed can reconnect. We used to think it was nearly impossible for those pathways to reconnect. Wonderful new research is being done in this area. The late notable Christopher Reeves, who was paralyzed as a result of an accident, lent much of his time and talents to assist ground breaking research in the area of spinal cord injuries.

Along with certain remembrances, Courtney's emotions become transparent again. She was able finally to grieve her losses and was able to shed tears. She began to remember little things that Zachary had said or done. She has been able to write poetry about him and to mention his name in conversation. Here is one of the poems she was able to write about Zak. It was placed in the newspaper on the first anniversary of his death.

It is often said that angels never age.
That is why you will always be
A sweet little boy with a twinkle in your eye, a smile
    on your face, a song
On your lips.
That is why we will always be lost without you.
Missing a part of our hearts that you once filled.
Missing your laughter and your smiles, your joyful
    outlook on life.
Your wide-eyed wonder at each moment.
Time will never ease the pain. It will never get any
    easier living without you. We will always love
    you.
                    Love,
                        Mom, Jerry, and Christina

She and Jerry erected a small, white, wooden cross at the accident site and decorated it for special occasions. One time, they had placed an Easter basket filled with toys, and as they were driving by, they saw a little boy carrying off the basket. Courtney said she felt good about this.

I've never liked the crosses simply because they are painful reminders, but I do know they comfort many people. I also know that my eyes always go to them whenever I'm driving. Fleeting questions of whom and what flash through my mind as I see those crosses, and I do tend to check my speed. Apparently these memorials do for others what they do for me. They cause me to pause, to slow down, and to consider that a lost life is represented here.

Our newspaper recently carried a feature article about these roadside memorials. The beginnings of such a practice are unknown, but these memorials have proven meaningful for those surviving. Many families feel so helpless after a traumatic loss, and the erection of a cross, a tree, or some kind of marker helps ease this desolation. The memorials become important in the grieving process of survivors. I notice also that now names are appearing on the crosses; this seems to lend more reality.

I recall that after the death of my children's father, a tree was planted on the Indiana University Campus in Bloomington, Indiana, in his honor. They have revisited this site, which I believe brings some comfort.

As grief stricken as all the family was, we never thought of being unforgiving of Courtney for her part in the tragedy. That's how it came to be for us—a tragic accident, a very tragic accident that any of us would have given almost anything for it never to have happened.

It took much longer for Courtney to forgive herself, I'm sure. Knowing every event in our life has spiritual significance and that even this event had been God-filtered must have helped ease her burden. God's forgiveness and grace have covered and still cover this whole situation. His mercy is freely given and if He does not keep score of our wrongs, why should we? I am aware that sometimes we do not feel this assurance. This is when we ask the Spirit to remind us that God's grace is not a matter of how we feel, but of what God has done for us. Whether we feel it or not, God's grace is ours.

The quote from Goethe seems fitting here: "It's the nature of grace always to fill spaces that have been empty." What a blessing!

We had to trust something good would come to us. Our job was to allow the experience to be used. It's not what happens to us that gives content to our lives, but whether or not we let the experience sink into our being in a positive way. No matter how complex or tragic our experience, God calls believers to reconciliation. Without reconciliation, bitterness reigns. This sounds like a platitude, but it is something that I am still learning to incorporate into my life. My hope and prayer is that, in time, complete restoration will come to the many wounded of this tragedy.

Courtney's new, stronger personality has helped her live with the fact that her daughter Christina is not with her. When this reality becomes painful, Courtney deliberately tries to focus her mind on all the positive things that she and Christina share. They talk on the phone weekly, see one another about every ten weeks, and correspond. Their times together are filled with laughter. No, it is not the same as having your child in your home, but it is having a child and having one who seems to be showing real strength of character for all that she has been through. It's focusing on what you have rather than what you've lost.

Six years is a short life to have lived on this earth, but Zachary left us a lasting legacy. A step grandfather, a few months before Zachary died, had developed a special relationship and understanding with Zachary that was not there before. Looking back, we know that God arranged this time of bonding before the end. A big stepbrother cherished feelings of tenderness that he had never felt before as he remembered roughhousing with Zachary. An older sister had realized that her little brother wasn't so bad now that he was school age. A book is birthed. A father had a son. Mothers remember.

CHAPTER SEVEN

THE INCREDIBLE HAPPENED

Our families were beginning to breathe a little easier. Courtney had been out of the hospital almost three months; she was progressing and things were falling into a manageable routine. Then the incredible happened. The Fayette County Prosecutor brought legal charges against Courtney.

Why such charges were pursued seemed unbelievable. We did not understand. I had been told by my lawyer in Bloomington that in our county such charges would never have been brought. Everyone involved had already suffered so much. Courtney herself had been through more pain than any mother should have to endure. Couldn't they see that the old Courtney had died in the accident? This new woman was a different person who did not even remember the accident. What justice is served in such a case?

Art had lost a son. Jerry had lost a stepson, almost a wife. Christina lost the family she knew. I felt immense sorrow. Our whole family grieved. We all knew that these legal charges were not going to bring Zachary back and only served to compound our heartache and strain fragile family relations. I could not believe it was happening.

Courtney was arraigned before a Fayette County Grand Jury in April of 1998. A Grand Jury was called because of difficulty in making a decision about the case. She was charged with reckless driving while under the influence of alcohol and causing a wrongful death.

On the advice of Jerry and her lawyer, Courtney pleaded guilty. Given all the circumstances, they felt this was the best decision. By doing so she avoided the trauma of a jury trial, but relinquished the right to appeal. All mercy would be upon the judge when sentencing came.

She was thirty two years old and only weeks out of her acute hospitalization. Her cognitive skills were still impaired at this time, and in fact, she was only just beginning on her road to recovery. I know she did not understand what was happening. Everything just seemed all wrong to me, and I could do nothing to make it right. I have never felt so powerless.

The next year and a half of waiting for sentencing required fortitude. Those eighteen months caused us all, especially Courtney, to look deep within for strength beyond ourselves. Except for the mercy and grace of God, I do not know how she or Jerry made it, for I knew how I was struggling. We did make it and, without a doubt, know it was God's strength within us.

During the waiting period, Courtney had many medical and psychological tests to determine her actual mental and psychological status. Her following letter (written just as she wrote it) shows just how hard this whole process was for her and how tense everyone was.

10-8-99

Dear Mom,

I am very sorry that I got so upset with you on the phone yesterday. This whole business with even having an MRI of my brain makes me very upset. And I've been having a very hard time since August. Since the accident I go down hill starting in August.

First it's Zak's birthday, then the day we had the accident, then the day he went to heaven.

This is a lot of things. Then I have the holidays to deal with.

Even Halloween makes me very sad. I dread the holidays now and want nothing more than for them to be over.

I always used to be so into the holidays, now I just go through the motions.

And there is no three time rule with the courts like I thought. (She was thinking that since this is her first offense, punishment would be lighter, I believe.)

The judge has the power to continue this for years. As bummed as that makes me feel I'm okay with it because I can go on with my life the best I can. Zak can't.

And if having my court stuff drag on more is what happens I feel like that's a bummer but at least I can have things drag on. Zak can't.

I do want to apologize again you did me a favor having Chris (our son-in-law who is a doctor) look at the MRI and I acted very nasty to you I'm sorry.

Love,
Courtney

There was one legal delay after another. Her lawyer was on a trip, the judge was busy, or papers weren't ready. Courtney and Jerry were brave during this time, but there came a point that we did not mention these legal issues, because there were no answers, and the game was 'wait.' None of us knew if, when, or whether Courtney would be sentenced and what that sentence would be. This waiting was one of our hardest tasks. Denial of the situation proved impossible. Family and friends wrote the judge on Courtney's behalf, hoping for leniency.

We took heart that other legal advice indicated she would not be sentenced. I hung my hope on this opinion. It was hard to imagine her being sentenced, given her emotional and physical condition at this time. I did not see how she could be adequately cared for in prison. It was hard enough to take care of her needs at home.

During these months of waiting, Courtney was allowed a trip to Denver to see her sister and brother-in-law, Julie and Ruben Federico. I accompanied her. I'll never forget the airport wheelchair trip; the funny, but scary, motorized shopping cart ride by Courtney through the aisles in Wal-Mart; the straw hat that she wore; the blossoms on the trees at Red Rocks; the feeling I had of helping my adult child, who was now disabled.

Courtney challenged Ruben to a hot pepper eating contest, never telling Ruben, who is Hispanic, that her taste buds had never returned. Guess who won? The memories of that trip will always remain with me. It was a precious time. Julie arranged nice events for Courtney: a soothing aromatic facial, times in the sun, a luncheon.

In spite of seeking after happiness, we all were aware of the cloud hanging over us. It cast a long shadow. Courtney had trouble eating and trouble sleeping. For the first time in my life, I took a pill for anxiety. Christina was not close by, but I'm sure she dealt with her own struggles at this time. Jerry's emotions were turbulent. Conrad and the rest of the children offered their best and remained strong with us.

During the wait, Conrad and I made some major life changes. We both not only retired, but in November of 1999, we moved to the town where I had grown up, still had family, and where we had investments. It was nice being only one hour from Courtney.

The day after we moved in, Courtney came to stay for a week since Jerry was going to Florida for a work conference, and he did not want to leave her alone. During that week, we had a special dinner for Courtney and invited her aunts, uncle, and cousins. Now we realize that being all together was a special gift. Little did we know that Courtney would be in prison by the next week. Looking back, I think how special and caring God was to give us this time together.

The sentencing date was set for November 28, 1999. The proceedings took place in adjacent Franklin County. On that day, Jerry, his mother, his aunt, Conrad, and I were with Courtney. Her lawyer was present. Courtney's counselor came to present expert testimony as to why Courtney was not emotionally stable to go to prison. I presented prayer to God the whole time. We listened and waited.

We found that the judge had not read the letters on Courtney's behalf, because he said they had not been copied to her lawyer. No one had told us to do this. That powerless feeling engulfed me again.

Without preliminaries, he sentenced Courtney to two years in prison and two years of probation for a Class C felony. She was convicted of reckless driving causing a wrongful death. A maximum sentence could have been sixteen years; he said he gave her the least possible sentence according to the law. We were very glad for this, but I didn't understand the legalities of handling a case in this manner. I would have thought he could have taken Courtney's physical and mental state into account as well as mitigating circumstances and maybe have sentenced her to only probation. Clearly, he was not sentencing the woman who had the wreck. She was gone; but the judge did not know.

It took about two minutes for the impact of the sentencing to penetrate our understanding.

Courtney's lawyer asked with disbelief, "You mean you are actually sentencing her?"

Clearly, we had thought it would not happen, or maybe we had just deluded ourselves into thinking that it would not.

The judge's resounding "Yes," and then his summarily leaving the chamber, left no doubt. We were plunged into disbelief. Courtney clung to Jerry and cried a cry that I will never forget.

"Oh, Jerry, they'll hurt me!"

She was obviously terrified of going to prison. We were all numb, some from fierce anger, all from searing pain. Our hearts were devastated. I am so thankful Conrad was there for me and just wrapped me in his protecting arms.

Courtney soon calmed down and so did I. I was able to give her a warm embrace before they took her away. I was so impressed with her strength at that moment and have been ever since.

From the courtroom Courtney was taken to the Franklin County Jail to await transfer to Indiana Women's Prison in Indianapolis, Indiana. I was so afraid for her emotional and physical well-being.

I was able to see her after a long 48 hours. She was dressed in the obligate, orange pant suit and looking pale and frightened but trying so hard to be courageous. I know she did not understand. We had to talk through a window glass and a telephone. The closest thing to touch was aligning our hands together on the glass pane. So close yet so far. A place I never dreamed of being.

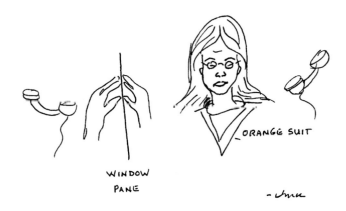

The county jail was not well-equipped to handle a disabled inmate. Courtney could not achieve a safe shower on her own because of the physical layout. The facility soon transferred her to Indianapolis Women's Prison.

Upon hearing Courtney's sentencing that cold November day, I wept. My mind refused the reality. We had all been so confident that the judge would see that she had already suffered as much as any mother could suffer. In legal eyes, though, wrong had been committed and accountability was demanded. The alcohol and drug charges were dropped, but a wrongful death had occurred.

The accident itself was just that: an accident. Zachary will not come back, nor will the old Courtney. None of our large and extended family will forget, but we can go on—with God's help. Courtney aches with regret for this tormenting mistake. She has had to pay legally with a part of herself that remembers forever.

CHAPTER EIGHT

BEHIND RAZOR WIRE: PRISON

I kept a journal of the prison months. The journal I kept is for me and others, because the story will never be told by Courtney.

She says, "All I want to say is that I spent time at the Indiana Women's Prison. I was charged with a class C felony. I was on a medical unit and I met some great ladies."

Volumes leap from these words. The nine months of my daughter's incarceration have been relegated to deep recesses of my mind, and I, too, only take out the memories reluctantly or if necessary.

I drew pictures of the high fences with razor wire. Most of the buildings were easily a hundred years old. What manner had these walls observed? The faces of the personnel could hold no warmth. At each visit I entered another world.

I described what an ordeal it was to see Courtney and the vexing rules once we managed to get into the visiting room. Pockets were emptied, coats locked up, signatures taken, and bodies scanned before we entered yet another locked door.

I visited alone or with Christina. I made it a point to see that Christina visited as often as possible. Christina's presence, while therapeutic, was bittersweet for Courtney. She wanted deeply to see her daughter but was embarrassed that her daughter was seeing her in prison. Christina seemed calm, but I wondered what was really going on in her young mind?

We were allowed two hugs only, one hug upon arrival and one on departure. Otherwise, there was to be no physical contact. No doubt it was a rule designed to curb transfer of contraband. There was to be no discussion except between you and your family, which could be no more than two visiting members. Courtney had put the names of only Jerry, Christina, and me on her visitors' list. Not even Conrad or Courtney's siblings could visit. She did not want anyone to see her in prison. Much later she added a few others' names.

The visiting area had a subdued atmosphere with family units speaking in hushed tones. Images remain forever in my mind. The sight of the very pregnant inmate was disturbing; the spectacle of small children visiting brought sadness to my heart. The soft words of a minister said to a pretty, young woman caused me to look away to give unavailable privacy. These are only a few of the haunting images.

Our visits became very intentional as we determined to find sunbeams in that place. We smiled and laughed more than other people in the room. It was rare to see smiles or to even hear laughter in the visiting room. We did have fun together on those unforgettable visits.

The Monks of New Skete in their book *Rise Up With a Listening Heart* tell us "Life is serious, but ... an insightful and healthy sense of humor is a defiant response to life's absurdities and challenges. Laughter carries... an energy that seizes despair and casts it overboard, re-establishing inner balance and calm. Through its own infectious rhythms, laughter spreads healing...." This fit for us.

We were allowed to take three dollars into the visiting room to buy drinks and snacks. I was so amused when Courtney said, "The machine coffee is so much better than coffee served at mealtime."

Courtney and I have always enjoyed quality coffee, and it was hard to imagine machine coffee as better than anything. Then I remembered that her taste buds had not returned.

Treats from the vending machine became almost an obsession for Courtney; her favorite was called Leopards, which was basically a Twinkie with artificial chocolate chips. Ohhhh.... Well, anyway, this ritual made for laughter and fun.

I didn't realize it then, but her obsession over the Leopards was a preview of her obsessive behavior to come.

Courtney spent nine long months in "Indianapolis," her preferred term. Nine months are needed to create new life. We have come to look on the Indianapolis nine months as the time Courtney needed to create her new life. The place became a watershed. She came back from the accident and Indianapolis a different woman.

Since the accident, both her short-term memory and a considerable amount of her long-term memory had been almost nonexistent. It was at Indiana Women's Prison in the summer of 2000, almost three years after the accident, that suddenly one day, Courtney said she knew that she had come out of the coma and she realized what had been going on in her life for the past three years.

I remember this epiphany. Her words were, "I have come out of the fog."

I am convinced God had kept parts of Courtney's memory unhealed while she was so physically and emotionally fragile. Otherwise, I don't think she would have survived. As she became stronger, she was given needed understanding. How beautiful, but imagine the bluntness of waking up and finding yourself in prison, behind high fences with razor wire.

****

The early prison months were a mental jumble for Courtney. The sensory overload nearly proved disastrous, until she learned to disengage by sitting on the sidelines, simply reading, doing cross-stitch, or remaining in her tiny room. Such activities allowed her private boundaries in her non-private world.

We were grateful Courtney was placed on a small, medical unit of 25 inmates rather than with the general prison population. I shuddered to think of her in the general prison population. Having a private room with an open window was an unexpected surprise. God must have known how she needed this small measure of privacy as well as the safety of a smaller unit. It took me some time to see God's hand in all of this, but it was there nonetheless.

Having a daughter imprisoned created new and unsettling emotions. I was closer than I wanted to be. Closer than I ever dreamed I would be. Prisons are a world apart. They are microcosms within a larger eco-system; a necessary evil of society with no obligation to serve families, which, in part, is understandable. As a family, though, we had found the rules and regulations surrounding telephone calls, visits, and sending money or packages akin to doing battle. The understandable need for regulations escaped us.

Phone calls from Courtney could only be collect, which was more costly. I know of cases where this expense precludes families from often talking to imprisoned loved ones. Calls were monitored, and during conversations this fact was announced every few minutes, which also increased cost. The fact that the lack of telephone privacy could feel so demeaning had never before entered my mind.

For security reasons, it's doubtful that the present prison telephone system can change. However, allowing inmates at least the ability to call toll-free 800 numbers (even with monitoring still in place) would ease a financial burden for families and inmates. Our phone bill was easily an extra twenty-five to thirty-five dollars per month, which is not a huge amount compared to Jerry's two hundred dollars a month bill.

Only two packages of specific dimensions could be sent to Courtney per month. Family members had to coordinate with Jerry, who was trying to mail Courtney her needed things. I remember Courtney's anxiety when I unintentionally mailed a package without going through Jerry. She didn't want anything to go wrong with the system's rules, because she wanted to make no waves, only to be invisible.

Courtney was allowed ten hours of visiting per month, and naturally she wanted Jerry to fill the majority of time. Christina and I usually visited monthly for an hour and a half. Only ten hours per month leaves many hours apart. Once I made the trip only to be told there was no visiting that day because of an official visit. One fellow inmate told Courtney that she had been there seventeen years and her out-of-state family had visited once. The loneliness can only be imagined.

As a result, mail became a lifeline for Courtney. Its importance is aptly expressed by an inmate when she was told that she was being prayed for, she asked for more letters instead. Letters become the connection to the outside world. Family and friends were so good to write. Courtney's identification number was on every letter. Letters received revealed a bright red, two-inch stamp indicating they had been mailed from a prison. I didn't care; I was thrilled to get her letters, and our mail lady, Teresa, gave no comments.

Through correspondence, Courtney started and renewed relationships with extended family members. My sister, Shirley, says she became soul mates with Courtney through those letters. Each letter was like a ray of hope to Courtney. From this experience, I will never forget how important letters are to those who are incarcerated.

Courtney wrote to keep her mind occupied and stimulated. Ever since regaining the ability to write after the accident, she has continued a never-ending correspondence with many people. It has become a ministry. At first, her penmanship was illegible because she had to write with her left hand since her right hand was paralyzed. Eventually, the computer proved a great writing friend. With time she has been able to regain use of her right hand.

Christina became the favored recipient of Courtney's writing. Even today Christina receives at least a daily postcard. Letters to her bear every imaginable sticker. Finally, the postman required a padded envelope for the sticks of gum. Through correspondence, e-mail, and phone calls, a precious long-distance relationship has continued between mother and daughter. This is appreciating what you have, not what you've lost.

We often take for granted freedoms like phone calls, mail, or just seeing someone, until these freedoms are taken away. Freedoms lost become dear. Even the freedom to enjoy color vanished, simply due to drab prison surroundings. Although she had never liked floral sheets, Courtney asked for those to brighten her little room.

At Indianapolis, Courtney developed a special friendship to a dear lady thirty years her senior. She and Maria (not her real name) shared confidences, and Maria, who had been in Indianapolis for seventeen years, became a mentor to Courtney. Among other things, she taught Courtney how to fold laundry as she thought Courtney needed improvement in this area. They began to share a love of recipes, and Maria volunteered her secret Hungarian Goulash dish. Collecting recipes became a mission as well as a salvation. Courtney and Maria had a new focus. Everyone sent Courtney recipes. She impresses me today with her boldness in trying new dishes. After serving twenty years, Maria was released. She and Courtney still write and share recipes.

Courtney kept to herself during this time in prison. Loneliness was preferable to being a part of the general discontent. She physically exercised every chance that she was given and walked outside for exercise, many times in the cold. She attended chapel services, participated in any craft opportunities, and did her best to keep a low profile and obey all the rules. She wasn't offered academic classes since she had her degree.

Courtney says, "It was nice to be able to do all of these things during the day, but at night I still had to go back to my 9x5 cell. The twenty-foot high fence with razor mesh on top was still outside of my window. I missed my family every night. I longed to have my husband lying beside me. I wanted to talk to my Mom, sister, and friends and know my conversation wasn't being recorded. I needed to see my daughter and be allowed to touch her. There were so many things I had taken for granted when I was free. I made a vow to myself and God that I would never again do anything against the law. The cost had been too high for me and my family."

Courtney's behavior did not go unnoticed. She was given a rare opportunity to be released three months early because of exemplary behavior. Maria told her she had been there seventeen years and had never seen this occur. On September 2, 2000, Courtney returned to the Franklin County Jail and three days later was home. She still faced two years probation.

 Nine months are needed to create a new life. After nine months our wife, mother, and child were returning to us a new person. What was she destined to do with this new life?

Courtney will never forget Indianapolis, but says only, "I want to put it behind me."

I want to put it behind me also.

Courtney survived prison, but it is an experience to be avoided. Although she faced two years of probation, she was now free to return home and begin her life again. She had paid her legal debt with a high price.

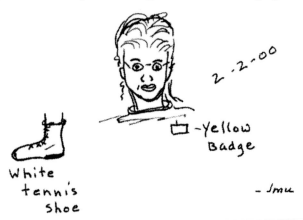

Courtney at Indianapolis 2-2-2000

CHAPTER NINE

"I CAN'T REMEMBER ME"

— COURTNEY —

My husband tells me that I am different now, but "I can't remember me." Mom says that my personality is changed, but I don't remember my other personality. I have had to get acquainted with the new me. I do know that I now have new physical disabilities. I do know that I have new obsessive behavior habits. Most of all, I know that I am very thankful to be alive.

I don't remember much about my prior personality, but from what little I do and from what people say, I must have been nervous, sometimes depressed and unsure of myself. My present nervousness comes from the compulsions that I have as a result of the brain injury. I am never depressed now, other than an occasional blue day. This, in itself, is wonderfully surprising. People today tell me I am very strong in my preferences of just about everything! This is a big change.

Is this new person really me? My main frustrations now are when I am doing something requiring physical ability or when I am dealing with my new compulsions.

At first, when I was wheelchair bound, I remember hating to ask people to take me to the bathroom. I understand that at Hook's Rehabilitation I had to go through a complete bladder retraining process. I just did not like being unable to do for myself. Many of you can identify, I am sure.

I hated Jerry's having to help me with my shower. He tried and did his very best, but it is not the same as being able to wash yourself. I remember his wrapping my leg cast in plastic to keep it dry. Later, I resented having to use a shower chair, but decided that if my 65-year-old mother-in-law didn't complain at having to use one, I wouldn't either.

Even today, I have to concentrate on walking to be able to walk right. I have to make myself think "heel, toe, pick up foot, keep head up." These things still aren't as automatic as they should be. I walk with a limp, which affects my stability. I often use a cane when in public. I need assistance of a rail to do stairs confidently. In my journal on 4-08-01, I wrote "Went to the dentist by myself. The stairs did not bother me." That felt good.

I suffered a severe, traumatic brain injury and many broken bones when involved in a car accident in which my six-year-old son Zachary died. The emotional center of my brain was greatly traumatized. It is only a miracle that I am alive and that my emotions have survived and returned at all.

The Brain Injury Association of Pennsylvania has an informative brochure that defines a traumatic brain injury (TBI) as an insult to the brain, not of degenerative or congenital nature, but caused by an external physical force that may produce a diminished or altered state of conscious, which results in an impairment of cognitive abilities or physical functioning. It can also result in the disturbance of behavioral or emotional functioning. I fit every detail of this description.

I have learned that I am not alone in my injury. Data from the Center for Disease Control relate the following incidence of brain injury in the year 2000:

— One and a half million Americans sustain a traumatic brain injury each year.

— Each year 80,000 Americans experience the onset of long-term disability following TBI.

— More than 50,000 people die every year as a result of TBI.

— The risk of TBI is highest between adolescents and young adults.

Data from the Brain Injury Association of America indicate that an estimated 5.3 million Americans live with some type of disability from Traumatic Brain Injury. This is roughly 2 percent of our population.

The following chart from the Center for Disease Control data shows the percentages of traumatic brain injury causes. My car accident places me in the transportation category, which is the largest cause of traumatic brain injuries.

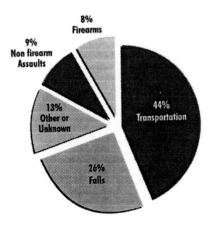

As shown below, the brochure also does a fine job of listing the consequences of brain injury:

THE CONSEQUENCES OF BRAIN INJURY

Cognitive Consequences Can Include:
- Short term memory loss
- Slowed ability to process information
- Trouble concentrating or paying attention for periods of time
- Difficulty keeping up with a conversation; other communication difficulties such as word finding problems
- Spatial disorientation
- Organizational problems and impaired judgment
- Unable to do more than one thing at a time
- A lack of initiating activities; or once started, difficulty in completing tasks without reminders

Physical Consequences Can Include:
- Seizures of all types
- Muscle spasticity
- Double vision or low vision, even blindness
- Loss of smell or taste
- Speech impairments such as slow or slurred speech
- Headaches or migraines
- Fatigue, increased need for sleep
- Balance problems
- Paralysis

Emotional Consequences Can Include:
- Increased anxiety
- Depression and mood swings
- Impulsive behavior
- More easily agitated

- Egocentric behaviors; difficulty seeing how behaviors can affect others

I find I relate to all three areas: cognitive, physical, and emotional consequences. It has taken a long time to make progress in these areas. I know I will never be the person I was before, but I do have my life. I have decided to strive to make it my best possible life.

My emotional journey has felt very strange. Few understand what it feels like to have no emotions over things about which you should have emotion. I realized my son was dead because I had been told, but all dead meant to me was "not alive anymore." I couldn't put any emotion behind this reality. I felt like a cold person. I did know enough to feel this. It's been more than eight years since my accident. In the past three years I have begun to put emotions behind the word "dead" and to realize that dead really means more than not alive.

At first, when I didn't have any emotions, I didn't do anything except read and write letters. This was my capability. I didn't always retain what I read, but I just kept reading and writing letters. My early letters were nearly illegible, because I had to use my left hand since my right hand was paralyzed. I think that my handwriting has improved over the years, and I am now able to use my right hand. I also retain much of what I now read.

After a lot of timidity, I can use the computer and this makes writing so much easier. I've even become enamored with e-mail and use it daily. I like being able to have this connection with people since my opportunity to travel is limited.

I couldn't cry more than a tear or two until the summer of 2001. At this time, I felt my first real emotions since before the accident. Now, more than eight years after the accident, I can feel what I call full force emotions. Jokingly, I told Mom that I "liked it better when I didn't feel so much emotion!" In reality, I am thankful, because many head injury victims never regain an appropriate emotional state, particularly when injured, as I was, on both sides of the brain.

It was not until two months after the accident that I was able to scrawl a few wobbly words on a journal page. Below are my very first attempts. I was at Hook's Rehabilitation Hospital on December 5, 1997.

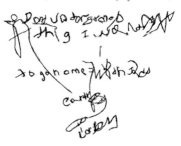

12-5-97 (Translation) I am very confused. I don't know what has happened to me or ... (end of entry). ...I want to go to Jerry. I'm so confused. I don't want to be confused anymore.

12-16-97 I'm not so confused...but I want my boy.

Courtney's Signature:

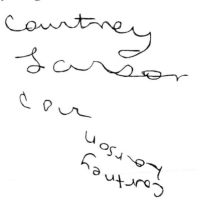

My Christmas message to Mom is written below. See the improvement in my writing?

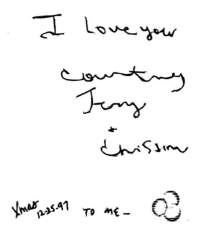

It wasn't until the summer of 2000, while I was an inmate at Indiana Women's Prison, that I began to be "unconfused" and to realize what had gone on in my life for the last three years. I had finally understood with some degree of feeling that I had been in a car accident, which had messed me up and taken the life of my little son. I suddenly also realized that I was in a prison but didn't understand why. Jerry had to explain all the legal aspects to me.

I was released soon after coming out of my fog. Since then I have been trying to become better acquainted with the new me. I am trying to rebuild my present life on those things I have rather than on what I have lost. I can say that God has been gracious.

I still remembered some things about my old self and sometimes felt that I was trying to fit that person into my new and different body and mind. It wasn't easy and often confused me at first. I wondered who I really was.

Though I can't remember my personality of years past, I am getting to know this person I now call "myself." My mother and my daughter are getting to know me and so are other family members. I find I like her. My husband likes her. She is my supreme second chance in life. Not everyone is given a second chance in life; I feel special. I still wonder at times why I was spared and not Zachary. God has helped me put aside survivor's guilt, but often professional help is needed to get through some of these hurdles.

CHAPTER TEN

WAYS I'VE FOUND TO LIVE AGAIN

— COURTNEY: 2003—

I am very happy with how I have surpassed medical expectations, but I know all the credit really goes to God. He kept me from dying. He has allowed me an incredible journey back, and He keeps my faith and hope just stretched enough that I persevere. Had I returned the same Courtney, I know I would not have had the emotional or physical strength to deal with the many, many issues facing me.

In the beginning, I did not have the physical stamina to do housework, and Jerry had to do everything. I am now able to cook and clean. I never knew it would feel so good to do dishes. I enjoy keeping our home and think it is so funny, because I know that before I had not liked cooking or cleaning at all. Another positive to my brain injury!

The whole arena of cooking is a new world to me. It began in Indianapolis when Maria and I, to stay occupied, started talking recipes. I've made things that I never dreamed I could or would even want to make. I'm proud of my squirrel dumplings, my carrot cake, and my chicken fiesta. I have begun to collect cookbooks. I'm actually learning how to use various spices.

Don't misunderstand me; it is still a major undertaking for me to make one of these dishes, but I am so happy that I can. I'm very slow, have my failures and have to throw things out, but Jerry is quite proud of my new cooking skills, too. They offer a nice change from his fried egg sandwiches.

My present compulsive behavior is my biggest challenge. I nearly drive myself crazy with these confounding compulsions. I think a lot of it is that I, for some reason, do not want to make a mistake, and this fact in itself is unusual for me. I just can't check something once and tell myself it's done right. I have to keep going back and checking and rechecking, which gets old, I can tell you.

Every now and then, my checking and rechecking pay off. One day I was examining my mail to make sure I had remembered everything, and in one envelope I had forgotten to enclose the letter! I know most people do note these things, but I have to check several times, and it's very frustrating. I always find myself still looking, even as I walk to the mailbox.

If I go out to feed the dog, I have to unlock both doors and observe, at least twice, that they are unlocked before I can walk outside. When I'm going to the store, I have to look in my wallet for money and a grocery list about five times.

As troublesome as the compulsions are, they are better than when I first came home from the hospital. I've learned tricks like making lists, trying to keep my life as simplified as possible, asking for help, keeping rested, and talking to my head. All of these help to some degree. In reality, though, this is an aftermath of my injury and one with which I must live. If the compulsions become really bothersome, medication may help, but at this point I want to do it on my own. I am just thankful that I can make some decisions.

One amusing thing is that when I make a mistake, many assume it is because of my injury and not just human error. I could take advantage of this, couldn't I?

Drinking liquids still challenges me. I choke easily and often have to remind myself to "tuck and swallow," as they taught me in the hospital. This may be the result of damage to my throat muscles from the tracheotomy and/or ventilator. I've just learned to live with it, and "tuck and swallow" has become another inside joke of the family.

Dr. Glen Johnson, in his book that I will mention in the next chapter, says that one important predictor of how well brain-injured people do depends on their sense of humor. If people can make jokes about themselves, he feels this is a very positive sign. I certainly did not appreciate Mom's early attempts at humor, but as I've healed, I've learned the value of humor. The other day on the phone, we spent good long-distance money laughing ourselves silly over the fact that I feel compelled to give too much information when asked a simple question. Some brain-injured persons do not have a normal social shut-off valve and give far too much information. I am definitely working on this compulsion.

I deal with pain on a daily basis in my left leg, ankle, and foot. It could be arthritis brought on by the complicated break in that leg. I've found that, along with medication, a frequent change of shoes seems to give relief. So it's nothing for me to change shoes every hour or two. I had some high top tennis shoes, which were my favorites. I called these my training shoes. They were so comfortable that I wore them until they fell apart. I called "time for training shoes" once too often. We've made these words into another spirit-lifting phrase also.

This ongoing pain has taken adjustment. I can really empathize with those experiencing chronic pain. To deal with my pain as well as my emotions, I play this little mental game with myself.

Each morning I'll say, "Okay, Head, you have ten minutes to feel sorry for yourself."

After that, I tell myself to feel better. And I do! I am so fascinated that this works, because the old Courtney needed medication to feel better. My pain is helped most by working out on my exercise equipment every morning without fail. I have to keep my body as limber as possible to keep my pain manageable. I also have to take high doses of ibuprofen and glucosamine.

I remember one day that my physical frustrations got the best of me as I tried and tried to untangle a wind chime hanging on my front porch. My fingers and brain just could not work together to straighten the mess. I was in tears until I jerked myself together and realized, "Now, Courtney, those truckers barreling down the highway out there really don't care whether this wind chime is untangled or not!"

That somehow helped me regain perspective. Quite frequently when I experience frustration, I just remember that the truckers really don't care.

Jerry and I and the whole family have tried hard to give humor its proper place, because we've found it so helpful. We allow phrases like "tuck 'n swallow," "time for training shoes," "I can't remember me," or "the truckers don't care" to pepper our conversation when we need a pick up.

I don't know why God chose to spare me, but I am going to make the best of each day, and I do always remember to thank Him. I have asked myself why Zachary died and not me, and I find no answers. I finally realized that when painful, unfair, or difficult things happen to us, it is not ours to ask why, but only ours to accept. I've learned that no matter what does or does not happen to me, God is always with me.

An acquaintance of Mom's had a car wreck in which she and her two sons were severely injured, but survived. Her friends said, "Oh, God was surely with you."

"God would have been with me even if I had died, or if I had not had the crash at all," she replied.

He tells us that He will never leave us nor forsake us, (Hebrews 13:5 NIV), and I have found this so true on this return journey of mine. It took time to come to this acceptance of the sovereignty of God, and I'll confess that sometimes I still struggle, lash out, and ask why. That's our humanness. I have grown, though, and in spite of my physical and mental disabilities, I feel that I am a stronger person. Jerry and I look at every day as our day that God has chosen to give us.

I still feel sad that Christina hasn't been with me during her teenage years. I have missed a lot. I am so thankful, though, for the strength of character that she has shown. We have kept in close touch and appreciate our time when together. I don't allow myself to dwell on missing her or Zak. I just keep thinking of all the blessings I do have.

Each year I am finding I feel sadness around Zak's birthday and the day he died. I don't think this is too unusual. I don't want to forget him. Jerry and I try to do something special in remembrance at these times. We have placed his picture along with a poem that I wrote in our newspaper, released balloons, and decorated his roadside cross memorial. My family remembers him with planted flowers, a call to me, or a prayer.

Whenever I put together a new picture album, I tuck a picture of Zachary among the pages. These things have helped ease our pain. One of my poems is shown below.

In Memory of Zachary (ZAK) Paris

This year you would have been ten years old.
How we wish you were here to hold.
Our only consolation is that you are in a better place.
 But we still wish we could see your face.
Time goes on and things change.
But one thing remains the same.
How much we miss you.
A boy like you can never be replaced.

I try to fill each day with meaningful activities. I have my own personal meditation time; I exercise to ward off my physical pain; I clean; I do correspondence, and I work on cross-stitch or my jewelry. Or I may visit my neighbor. Often I will ride the rural transit into town to shop or for an appointment. Being able to negotiate the transit makes me feel good.

We visit Jerry's children and our grandchildren. The little ones bring us joy. I occasionally make a business trip with Jerry but always find this a challenge. We do attend local business and social functions. It is a real delight to be able to do some of these things, because for so long I could do almost nothing. I feel like I have a life again.

Sometimes I think I will try to drive again, but I am still hesitant. I'm not persuaded I have the needed judgment. I also think about working and hope that someday I will be able, because the desire to be productive is commanding. I was just beginning to put my college degree to work when the accident happened and sometimes have fleeting melancholy that all that effort can't be put to dynamic use. But then my life is not over yet . Who knows?

With Mom's help, I began to design and make jewelry. We order our supplies from the Internet. I make simple bracelets using Swarovski crystals and sterling silver clasps. I make each one an original design complete with a pewter star. This little star on the bracelet is called the "Zaky star" in remembrance of him.

At first I had great difficulty holding the crimping tool needed for attaching the clasp. The fine motor skills were more than I could do at the time. The first bracelet took me forever to make. I became frustrated, but did not want to give up, even though I felt like it. We have kept that first bracelet with all its imperfections. Mom just kept encouraging me. We have not aggressively marketed the bracelets, but I was happy when I sold a couple that I had displayed at Anne's, my friend's shop in Metamora, Indiana. Anne is the mother of Dr. Nathan Millikan, who visited me in the Cincinnati Hospital.

I've also branched out to making wine charms. Making the bracelets and the wine charms has helped fill that need and desire to be productive again. Both items may be ordered through my e-mail address and our web site, which are listed in the Selected Resources section at the end of the book.

I don't know what the future holds, but I do have faith that God will be there for me. The accident has affected each of us in a different manner and will continue to affect how we live our lives. I do think that we have all drawn closer as a family unit, which is good, for all too often tragedy pulls families and individuals apart. In another chapter, my family will relate how they have learned to live again.

Once I began to feel emotion again, or actually, once I came back to reality, I had to make a decision whether I was going forward after this experience or going backward into a state of chronic grief. With God's help, Jerry and Christina's help, and the help of the rest of my family, I decided to continue my new life's journey, to be there for my daughter, honor the memory of Zachary, and use my experience to help others. This effort is an ongoing process, but one in which I have found what I know is a purpose to live again.

Writing this book has been difficult for me and at first I did not want to do it. It resurrected too many painful memories. Mom needed to write to heal. I found that my desire was to share my story with others as encouragement. I don't like what I've been through, but maybe someone will be helped to carry on his/her journey.

CHAPTER ELEVEN

My Life with a Disability

— Courtney —

Jerry and I have tried to educate ourselves about head injuries and have found a helpful book to be Doctor Glen Johnson's handbook called *Traumatic Brain Injury Survival Guide*. This book is written for families and is easy to understand. His website is listed in the Selected Resources. Doctor Johnson is former clinical director of the Neuro Recovery Head Injury Program at Traverse City, Michigan. He has worked extensively with traumatic brain injury patients; the book is available electronically on his website. We found it a wonderful handbook and, with Dr. Johnson's permission (and Mom's help), I'll paraphrase some of its content.

He says that the brain weighs only three pounds but consists of more than 100 billion cells. To understand how the brain works, he uses the analogy of an orchestra in which there are different musical sections. All the sections must work together for beautiful music and all await the conductor for instruction. He says, for example, if the drum section hasn't been practicing, the overall sound of the music may be off. If an area of the brain has been injured, then the brain's overall performance may not be up to par or may not make good music.

Doctor Johnson reflects that, "While we once thought of the brain as a big computer, we now think it's like millions of little computers, all working together."

It's commonly known that the brain has two parts consisting of a right and a left hemisphere. Each side controls different things. Doctor Johnson says the right side deals with visual information and organizes or groups information together. The analytical left hemisphere takes this organized information and applies language to it.

For example, he says, the right hemisphere sees a house, but the left hemisphere says, "Oh yeah, I know whose house that is—it's Uncle Bob's house."

With a right-sided brain injury, important information usually does not get processed in the correct manner. In fact, a person may feel there is nothing wrong simply because the brain isn't processing correctly. A left-sided brain injury usually creates difficulty in problem solving or in more complex activities. The left side of the brain is also concerned with language and emotion.

My language ability remained nearly intact, which was not anticipated. My counselor said that because of this, the true severity of my injury was sometimes masked. At first, my speech was slow and halting because I wanted to enunciate every word in order to be understood. In the beginning, I found that talking exhausted me. I thought that I was unable to talk as fast as my brain could think, but in reality my brain was not making necessary connections.

I'm told that for many months after the coma, I spoke with an English accent, which my neurologist said was not unusual for post coma patients. The brain, it seems, has its own say about some things. My speech pattern was very stiff and formal, and I used words like "Mother" and "Daughter" instead of Mom or Christina. My regular accent finally did return. Mom says that I have a country twang and yes, that has returned. I had speech therapy and probably should have had more, but I feel I have made wonderful progress with my ability to talk. I do notice though that when I am physically tired, my speech ability declines as do my motor skills. My words begin to sound slurred and my walking becomes unsteady.

I had intracranial bleeds in both sides of my brain. I had a left-sided skull fracture, which caused further swelling and bruising. These are other ways the brain also may be injured. To monitor the swelling, the doctors had placed an intracranial pressure monitor. If increased pressure was noted, appropriate medicines were used to try to decrease the swelling and to preserve the integrity of the brain. I'm sure I looked frightful; my head was shaved and I had many cuts on my face, head, and arms. One head wound had staples. So much for glamour after a head injury!

I doubt I would have survived had I not received the aggressive treatment from the competent teams of the Intensive Care Surgery Trauma Unit of University Hospital at the University of Cincinnati, Ohio. I had so many great doctors whom I won't name for fear of omitting one. The nursing staff, my mother said, was also wonderful.

I'm told it was eleven days before I even opened my eyes, but I remember nothing until three months after the accident. Even then, and for several months after, things were still blurry. As I said, I didn't really wake up until the summer of 2000, almost three years after the accident. I have to accept what my family tells me about this period of my life. In truth, I'm glad that my full memory of this time will never return.

Doctor Johnson says that memory can be divided into immediate, short-term, and long-term memory. Immediate memory is where one is able to spit back information quickly. Johnson defines short-term memory as the ability to remember something about thirty minutes; long-term memory applies to information we are able to recall after a day, two weeks, or ten years.

Nearly everyone with a head injury has impaired memory. I did, and I still do. At first, I had almost no immediate or short-term memory. I could not be left alone and constantly was asking the same question. Even my long-term memory was quite faulty and is still not the best, but I have come a long way.

When I first awakened from the coma, I vaguely remembered Jerry, my daughter, mother, siblings, and other extended family members. I accepted that Jerry was my husband because he told me that he was, but I didn't remember having a husband. I recall waking up one morning after I was home and wondering who this strange man was. He said that I asked to see our marriage license and, as strange as it seems, the only signature I recognized was Zachary's scribbled print. Zachary and Christina had stood up with us at our wedding and had signed the license. It seemed I had a husband.

I soon remembered other close family members. But I still didn't remember much about Zachary as a person, much less as my son.

I had amnesia about events prior to the accident as well as events afterwards. Dr. Johnson says amnesia means losing a memory that you once had. Retrograde amnesia means losing memories prior to an accident. It's like a blackboard that's been erased; the more severe the head injury, the greater the retrograde amnesia. My last prior memory was of March, 1993, when my mother and stepfather came to my workplace to tell me of my dad's accidental death. This particular past memory probably remains because it is so significant, but there is so much even before this that I do not remember.

Loss of memory for events following an accident is called anterior grade amnesia. In my case, these memories also were erased, which is most likely due to the brain injury itself. At first, I could remember nothing of the accident and very little about Zachary. I still don't remember months of my hospitalization, but recently Jerry and I were talking about the accident. I told him that I remembered that I was going to hit the tree.

I have been able to face reality since it has returned in snippets. I really haven't been given more than I could handle at any one time. In my head I had always known this to be God's promise, but now I know it in my heart.

Little by little, in bits and pieces, some of my memories have returned as my brain has slowly healed. There is still much I cannot remember and may never. If I really think about it. Chunks of my life are all but erased from my memory.

CHAPTER TWELVE

THOSE CLOSEST SPEAK OUT

— JERRY —

My life changed completely as a result of the accident. My whole family was suddenly gone. My little stepson was dead, my stepdaughter living with others, and my wife's life hanging in the balance. I was lost. I won't deny that these were dark days. I struggled to keep it together. Many days I was unsuccessful, but somewhere from the depths of my inner being, I resurrected my relationship with God. I had long believed in God but was not close in my relationship with Him. In the depth of my deepest need, though, I found He met me again.

I soon realized that God was busily working to help me in my crisis. He used many people and many ways to do His work. My employer was very helpful in allowing me leave time. My fellow employees took up a financial contribution. Friends offered gifts of themselves and their time. I felt that we had the best of medical care, even during our times of misunderstanding with the medical system. Insurance, while it didn't cover everything, did care for most of the immense medical bills. I came to realize the great value of all these gifts.

I wanted to be with Courtney every possible moment and spent many hours and nights at her bedside. I didn't know if she would live, but I just felt that God could not take both of them. When I saw that Courtney was going to live, I knew she was spared because it was not her time. Knowing that she was spared has made us value the present. This also helps us bear the pain. So, I guess there really is a way through our sorrows if we will just look and believe.

Life is different now. Christina is gone. I can never get over the loss of Zachary, but I have a strong, precious wife. I have a job into which I've been able to pour energy and realize satisfaction. In my fifties, I have been able to finish educational goals begun years ago. These things now fill my life.

Helping Courtney regain independence has been my major goal and focus. In spite of everything, she is still Courtney to me. I encourage her to keep trying and to keep achieving. We try to laugh about some of the stuff, but I always want to be there for her. "It really doesn't matter" is one of our most helpful phrases.

Even though she thinks she never wants to drive again, I've encouraged her to drive the car around our acreage. She's ready to challenge the riding mower, I believe. I am proud of her new cooking skills as well as her courage to ride the rural transit into town and do some shopping by herself. She says it's more fun than shopping with me, since I dislike shopping anyway.

We keep working on the compulsions, but sometimes I just have to say to her, "Courtney, sit down! It doesn't really matter that the picture is crooked, that your shoes are not put away, or that piece of paper is lying there."

She has an excitement about things and events that she didn't exhibit before the accident. She seems to enjoy things more. This I find endearing. Maybe it's just that she values, in a new light, what she does have.

I know she misses Christina significantly, but she knows that by now Christina has adapted to her new environment and needs no further upheaval. They remain in close touch by phone, letters, e-mail, and when possible she visits every two or three months. The best, given the circumstances.

Five years ago, my oldest son Scott, and his wife Kathy, had their first child. She was my first grandchild. Courtney immediately ranked among the youngest step-grandmas around. Tessa, our granddaughter, has brought a new focus to our lives and fills a void.

Scott misses Zachary, because, as he said, "That little kid made me feel emotions I had never felt before." Scott and Zak enjoyed rough housing together.

Brandon, a grandson, has since come along and the void gets smaller all the time, even though we're aware that nothing will ever fill the empty space of Zachary and Christina.

All in all, Courtney and I are managing. I have more of a caretaking role than previously, but it's one for which I am thankful. We now take one day at a time.

Did it take all that we have gone through to arrive at this point of acceptance of our present lives? I don't know. I only know what I see and feel now. I have had to come to a realization that someone larger than me is in control.

— CHRISTINA —

Losing my little brother and having to move almost five hours away was the most difficult thing for me about the whole accident. My life changed.

It was very hard to start a new school, but I met a friend who was helpful to me in those early days of my new life.

On the positive side, I can say that I met many more new friends. I came out of my shell, so to speak, and talked more. I found a new church, became a Christian, and enjoyed being active in the church. I became involved in the youth group. I occasionally taught Sunday School to the children and sometimes sang with a group during church.

I became part of a big, noisy extended family. I had a big brother, a big sister, and a little sister. There were lots of pets. This helped fill up my life even though I missed my other family.

****

The following poem was written by Christina just one year after the accident. The poem was published in an anthology for young authors.

Young and Free

I am young and free and nothing can touch me
I wonder how the world will end and when
I hear the wind hitting the sides of the rocks
I see the huge sun looking back at me
I want for nothing more than what I have
I am young and free nothing can touch me

I pretend I can fly far away so when it comes I'll be
   safe
I feel the clean wind on my face
I touch everything I can

I worry about what will happen and what will be
I cry about things that make me sad
I am young and free and nothing can touch me
I understand that the world will end
I say I will beat it

I try to look for the good in what I see
I hope that the power of evil will not overtake me
I am young and free and nothing can touch me.

****

As a grandmother, I believe close observation reveals
a collage of invincibility, denial, and grief and yet, a
hope and feeling of resurrection. Youth grieve in the
ways of youth, but they need as much help in reconciling
their grief as do adults.

— Mother —

This experience came as a sudden shock. For the first two years, I could not even mention the accident without tears. I felt such loss and pain and wondered if I could make it through. But with God's outrageous grace and tincture of time, I have come to accept our new life. I am so very thankful for this new daughter. And she is a new daughter. We lost the old Courtney, as well as Zak, with the accident. I love Courtney's new strength and her personality. She makes us laugh.

Conrad and Courtney have begun to really enjoy one another's company. He finds her unabashed honesty refreshing. They have been known to send a thank you note for the thank you note! Courtney, Jerry, and Christina, are all inspirations to me. They haven't given up, so I can't think of giving up.

Christina has grown into a beautiful young woman, both inside and out. She exhibits strong, independent character with compassion. I feel a grandmother's pride. It could only have been through God's help, for things certainly could have gone otherwise.

I miss my grandson. He's still the six-year-old boy in my mind, yet I wonder what kind of individual he would be, what would his personality be like? God has given us a gift even though it is bittersweet. At our church there is a young boy who caused both Conrad and me to do a double take when we first saw him. He looked exactly like Zachary. We have gotten to watch Aaron (not his real name) grow these past few years and feel as if we have seen Zachary grow, too. This has been a heart-tugging experience, but nonetheless a gift from God.

We've all had to come to the realization that some lives are meant to be short upon this earth and that

Zachary's was one of those. We dwell upon what he left us rather than what we're missing. I still keep pictures of Zak around and find myself chuckling at the mischievous look he always had. He's always included in our number of grandchildren. The one who lives with Jesus. I keep him alive to the other grandchildren by mentioning his name and antics to them. Courtney tucks a picture of him among the photos of every album she makes.

I have just completed a photo album of nearly all the pictures I have of Zachary. I enjoy going through the album. It was actually made for Courtney and Christina, but in this way I remember him.

I feel that I can say that my grief over Zachary is now complete. I am recovered. It feels odd to say recovered because we don't usually associate recovery with grief, but I like this concept. Other sources talk about reconciling our grief. Whether we recover or reconcile, the important thing is that we learn to live with our grief. It will be a part of us forever after. Many of us, unfortunately, go through the rest of our lives with our recovery incomplete, probably because the recovery process is so hard. I have witnessed this and have seen the sadness of a life so affected.

I can face Zachary's birthday and his death anniversary with only a touch of sadness now. That feels so good. I spent time going through a program for moving beyond death and loss. *The Grief Recovery Handbook* by James and Friedman was helpful; the book is listed in the Selected Resources. Perhaps this book will be helpful to you also.

I do something in his remembrance on his special days. There will always be a space reserved for Zachary in my heart, but that is just the way it is when you have loved someone. This year I picked a huge bouquet of Montana wildflowers even including the pretty purple thistle. The thistle reminded me that at times Zachary could be prickly, too! I think that sometimes after we lose a loved one, we put them on a pedestal and soon forget that they were also human. I want to remember Zak's humanness.

I feel stronger for having gone through this experience. I can relate to people on many levels. More levels than ever I wanted. I still do not know why God led me through this valley, but I am determined to find all the good that I can gain from this journey and to let God use that for His glory.

There have been many occasions already to help others through similar pain. I have found that grief is one of the most common experiences of human beings and that feelings associated with grief are universal.

Perhaps the need to tell the story has been more necessary for me than for Courtney. It has been a humbling experience to share, but sharing has helped diminish my pain.

When it became dark enough, I could see the stars all shining and bright covering my head.

An old Chinese proverb says the same: "It's better to light a candle than to curse the darkness."

CHAPTER THIRTEEN

INFORMATION FOR FAMILIES

Unexpected deaths leave many secondary victims. It is estimated that each sudden and unexpected death affects 10 other people, which means more than 4,000 new secondary victims are created each day in our country as a result of accidents, suicides, and homicides.

There were 6,328,000 car accidents in 2003 with 2.9 million injuries. The cost for such accidents exceeds 230 billion dollars. Motor vehicle deaths stood at 42,643 in 2003; 17,013 or 40 percent of the deaths were alcohol related.

With sudden deaths, such as suicide, heart attack, or automobile accident, there is no such thing as anticipatory grief. There is only shock, which is why most of us need help through such a morass.

The following organizations, begun by the bereaved, seek to help the bereaved through difficult days associated with loss and grief. Many states also have associations concerned with preventing brain injury and improving quality of life for survivors and their families. The National Brain Injury office offers advocacy, education and support to families. I benefited from our state organization's support group.

Compassionate Friends and Bereaved Parents exist as survivors helping survivors. Their grassroots efforts have grown into national organizations. The same applies to Mothers Against Drunk Driving (MADD).

With Courtney's incarceration, I couldn't help but think also about prisoners' rights. I was pleased to learn about an organization called CURE, an acronym for Citizens United for Rehabilitation of Errants. CURE is a membership organization of families of prisoners, prisoners, former prisoners and other concerned citizens. The two main goals of CURE are: 1) to use prisons only for those who have to be in them, and 2) for those who have to be in them, to provide them all the rehabilitative opportunities they need to turn their lives around.

Co-founders and directors, Charles and Pauline Sullivan, organized a bus trip in 1972 to allow families of Texan prisoners the ability to travel to see their loved ones, many of whom they had not seen for more than ten years. This initial, successful trip led to monthly trips, then weekly bus trips. Soon bus trips were forming all over Texan cities, and one of the first organizations dealing with family and prisoner rights was born.

CURE grew to focus on advocacy as well as services. The organization was among the first grassroots efforts to look at what eventually became comprehensive prison reform. Numerous proposals were introduced to the Texas legislature aimed at prisoner rights. Many states now have chapters of CURE.

CURE takes a position on prisoners' telephone charges. They advocate that prisoners should have a debit card or prepaid calling card, and that prisoners should be allowed to call 800 numbers on their PIN lists.

Also, CURE feels that in the case of collect calls, the recipient should be able to select the carrier (billed party preference) and that there should be no surcharge. These were my feelings exactly.

In many states, relatives of prisoners pay much more for the collect calls from prisoners than would be paid on the outside for equivalent calls. In New York, for example, on average, they pay about 66 percent more (source: www.curenational.org web site). In many states the Department of Correction receives a commission from telephone companies. This amounts to huge amounts of money paid by prisoners' relatives.

I have contended that family support and contact are very important to the prisoner. Courtney has said that the mail and the phone were her lifelines while in prison. These excessive phone costs effectively isolate prisoners and deteriorate family relationships.

Others are beginning to be more open about their loved ones behind bars. For so long it was a subject unmentioned. In the November 22, 2004, issue of *People's Magazine*, a mother speaks out about her imprisoned son. Ms. Sherry Grace has begun a nonprofit group called Mothers of Incarcerated Sons. She has helped 1300 men in 23 states thus far. She helps find jobs for paroled inmates. She offers services to families; she has persuaded wardens to move inmates closer to home, and she has lobbied for mandatory minimum sentence guidelines.

In this article entitled "Hearts Behind Bars," she says her job is to be cheerleader, confidant, and crusader. She wants every mother of an incarcerated son to know she is in her corner. She says people tend to think that someone is a failure when he goes to jail. She feels this is a wrong attitude and that failure is only temporary. I find such views refreshing, and I think that such articles will help break down the stigma of having a loved one behind bars. Concrete but basic help is what is needed for families.

Knowing about these organizations and contacting some of them was very helpful to me. I hope they may be helpful to you also. So many kind people are willing to share their pain, as someone shared with them. In this way we are healed.

EPILOGUE

Courtney and Jerry still reside in Laurel, Indiana. Courtney stays busy with being mother and grandmother, her cooking, and craft projects. She continues to write. Jerry remains her loyal supporter and husband.

Christina has attended college and is currently working.

Judy and Conrad continue to keep Muncie, Indiana, as home base. Judy continues to enjoy retirement, her family, and writing.

Both Courtney and Judy are available for inspirational speaking at churches, groups, and organizations.

— APPENDIX —
SELECTED RESOURCES

BOOKS:

Traumatic Brain Injury Survival Guide by Dr. Glen Johnson, Clinical Neuropsychologist, former Clinical Director of the Neuro Recovery Head Injury Program, Traverse City, MI, 49684.

Love, Greg & Lauren by Greg Manning; Bantam, NY, NY, 2002.

Do They Have Bad Days in Heaven? by Michelle Linn Gust, M.S.; Bolton Press Atlanta, Roswell, GA, 2001.

The Grief Recovery Handbook by John W. James and Russell Friedman; Harper Perennial, NY, NY, 1998.

Healing After Loss by Martha Whitmore Hickman; Harper Perennial, NY, NY, 2002.

When a Friend Dies, A Book for Teens About Grieving and Healing by Marilyn E. Gootman; Free Spirit Publishing, Minneapolis, MN, 1994.

ARTICLES:

"Hearts Behind Bars by Sherry Grace," *People's Magazine*; Nov. 22, 2004.

"Resolution Versus Reconciliation: The Importance of Semantics" by Alan D. Wolfelt, Ph.D., Director, Center for Loss and Life Transition, Fort Collins, Colorado.

Bible references are taken from the *New International Version,* published by Zondervan.

Permission granted by Christina N. Paris for use of poem "Young and Free."

Permission granted by Dr. Alan Wolfelt to quote from his article "Resolution Versus Reconciliation: The Importance of Semantics."

Permission granted by sculptor Charles Schiefer to picture the Zaky Bear.

ORGANIZATIONS/WEB SITES

Brain Injury Association of America
8201 Greensboro Dr. Suite 611
McLean, VA 22102
703-761-0750
web site: http://www.biausa.org
e-mail: family helpline@ biausa.org or 1-800-444-
6443

Mothers Against Drunk Driving
National Office:
511 E. John Carpenter Frwy. Suite 700
Irving, TX 75062
1-800-438-6233
Fax: 972-869-2206/07
web site: http://www.madd.org/home/

CURE (Citizens United for Rehabilitation of Errants)
P.O. Box 2310
National Capitol Station
Washington, D.C. 20013-2310
202-789-2126
web site: http://www.curenational.org

The Compassionate Friends
P.O. Box 3696
Oak Brook, IL 60522-7696
630-990-0010
Toll free: 877-969-0010

Organ and Tissue Donation
Best to use Google.com as a search engine

American Foundation for Suicide Prevention
120 Wall Street, 22nd Floor
New York, NY 10005
212-363-3500
web site: www.asfp.org

Other Web Sites:
Tami Briggs, Harpist; Therapeutic Music
PO Box 62511
St. Louis Park, MN 55426
www.musicalrelections.com/home.cfm

web site for Dr. Glen Johnson: www.tbiguide.com

web site for Kids Who Are Grieving:
www.freespirit.com

web site for Judy Martin-Urban:
www.judeurbanski.com

E-MAIL ADDRESSES

Courtney's e-mail: jlarson9@aol.com

Judy's e-mail: Urbanski4u@aol.com

Dr. Glen Johnson's e-mail: debglen@yahoo.com

JUDY MARTIN-URBAN

Judy Martin-Urban resides with her husband Conrad in her home-town of Muncie, Indiana. Their blended family includes eight children and seventeen grandchildren.

Judy received her Masters in Women's Health from Indiana University/Purdue University of Indianapolis. She practiced in Women's Heath and taught nursing for many years. She has published articles, coauthored an e-book on real estate, and is currently writing an inspirational romance.

email address: Urbanski4u.com@aol.com

web site: www.judeurbanski.com

Courtney Martin Larson

Courtney Martin Larson graduated from Indiana University in criminal justice and public affairs. She is mother to 21-year-old Christina. She and her husband Jerry live in Laurel, Indiana. Courtney enjoys exercising, cross stitching, cooking, gardening, reading and a correspondence ministry. She makes Swarovski crystal bracelets and wine charms, each having a "Zaky star" in honor of her son Zachary, who died in the accident.

email address: jlarson9@aol.com

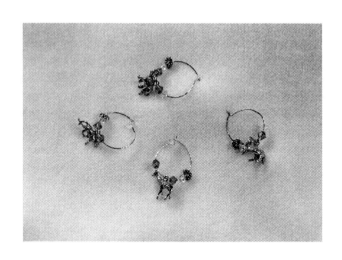

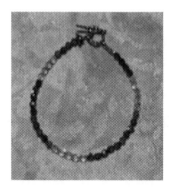

SWAROVSKI CRYSTAL BRACELETS

FOR INFORMATION:
Email: jlarson9@aol.com

ZAKY JEWELRY ORDER FORM

Date: _____

Name: _____

Address: _____

City, State: _____ Zip: _____

Phone: _____ Email: _____

BRACELETS — $10 EACH   COST

Quantity: ___ @ $10 each $ _____
Color of Stone: _____ Tax: _____
                         S/H: $1.50 ea.   _____

                         Subtotal $ _____

WINE CHARMS — SET OF FOUR (4) FOR $12.00

Quantity: ____ @ $12 per set $ _____
                         Tax: _____
                         S/H: $1.50 set   _____
                         Subtotal: _____

                         Total: $ _____

Mail Check or Money Order to:
Courtney Larson
P. O. Box 3296
Muncie, Indiana 47307
765-698-2148

E-mail jlarson9@aol.com

Orders shipped 1-2 weeks unless supplies backordered

— To Order —

I Can't Remember Me
by Judy Martin-Urban and Courtney Martin Larson

If unavailable at your favorite bookstore,
LangMarc Publishing will fill
your order within 24 hours.

— Postal Orders —
LangMarc Publishing
P.O. Box 90488
Austin, Texas 78709-0488
or call 1-800-864-1648
or online www.langmarc.com

I Can't Remember Me
USA $12.95 + $2.50 Postage
Canada: $16.95 + $5 Postage

Send _____ copies of _I Can't Remember Me_

_____

_____

_____

_____

Phone: _____

Check Enclosed: $ _____

Credit Card # _____
Expires: _____